Medical

An **Instant** Translator

Medical Spanish

An **Instant** Translator

Isam Nasr, MD, FACEP

Assistant Professor, Department of Emergency Medicine,
Rush Medical College;
Attending Physician, Department of Emergency Medicine,
Cook County Hospital,
Chicago, Illinois

Marco Cordero, MD, FACEP

Assistant Professor, Department of Emergency Medicine,
Rush Medical College;
Attending Physician, Department of Emergency Medicine,
Cook County Hospital,
Chicago, Illinois

Foreword by
Robert R. Simon, MD, FACEP

Professor and Chairman,
Department of Emergency Medicine,
Rush Medical College and Cook County Hospital,
Chicago, Illinois

W.B. SAUNDERS COMPANY
A Division of Harcourt Brace & Company
Philadelphia London Toronto
Montreal Sydney Tokyo

W.B. SAUNDERS COMPANY

A Division of Harcourt Brace & Company

The Curtis Center
Independence Square West
Philadelphia, PA 19106

Library of Congress Cataloging-in-Publication Data

Nasr, Isam.
    Medical Spanish : an instant translator / Isam Nasr, Marco Cordero;
foreword by Robert Simon. — 1st ed.
      p.   cm.
    ISBN 0–7216–6052–5
    1. Spanish language—Conversation and phrase books (for medical
personnel)   2. Medicine—Terminology.   I. Cordero, Marco.
II. Title.
    [DNLM: 1. Medicine—phrases—Spanish.   W 15 N264m 1996]
PC4120.M3N38   1996
468.3′421′02461—dc20
DNLM/DLC   95–39974

MEDICAL SPANISH   ISBN 0–7216–6052–5

Printed in the United States of America

Last digit is the print number: 9 8 7 6 5 4

The authors dedicate this book to their families.

Foreword

Rarely has there been a medical Spanish pocket manual that is as user-friendly as this manual. The authors have "field tested" their work among residents and faculty, as well as in courses taught by the authors. The physicians who utilized this manual on a trial basis were impressed with its uniquely practical design and approach. Common presenting complaints are organized using a logical combination of organ system and anatomical chapter headings. Thus, abdominal and genital urinary complaints are covered in the same chapter, since the physician seeing a patient with complaints related to gastrointestinal and/or genital urinary problems is often required to ask questions related to both systems.

Anatomical terms are arranged alphabetically, with both the Spanish word and the proper pronunciation—once again a unique concept that the authors have devised. You can look up virtually any anatomical term in the first few pages of the book and find the Spanish word as well as how to pronounce it to the patient.

The next chapter covers common phrases used by the physician seeing a patient in his or her clinic or in the emergency department. Phrases such as "is there someone with you who speaks English" or "speak slowly" are phrases that one wishes were available when seeing a patient. Other manuals that require a physician to look up individual words are inappropriate for the clinical setting. Phrases such as "what is the problem" or "where does it hurt" are rarely found in Medical/Spanish manuals. Another section instructs patients on how often to take medication, whether to take it before bedtime, and to avoid alcohol. Miscellaneous terms such as phlegm, faint, and burning are also listed. Even sections indicating cardinal numbers up to 100 and instructions used by triage personnel asking for the patient's name, phone number, and age are included.

The chapters, arranged according to patients' chief complaints, ask relevant questions and have been compiled based on a review of the authors' actual cases, in which they have detailed all of the questions they would ask a patient presenting with a complaint. These are all organized with the English question in the left column and the corresponding Spanish question, as well as pronunciation, in the right column. This is followed by common phrases such as "open your mouth" used during an examination and, finally, discharge instructions, including common specific instructions such as "take one antibiotic (penicillin) tablet every six hours."

The authors have produced a truly exceptional, easily usable pocket manual that should be a part of every physician's clinic or emergency department. It is the medical Spanish equivalent of antibiotic pocket manuals or interpretations of laboratory tests. This manual is truly unique and has been field tested—I recommend it to all physicians.

Robert Simon

Preface

Language barriers often impede good medical care. In daily practice, health care providers depend on their communication skills to obtain pertinent medical information. In many cases these skills are hindered when caring for non–English-speaking patients, thus compromising the quality of patient care. Hispanics are projected to become the largest minority group in the United States by the year 2000; as the Spanish-speaking population increases, it becomes paramount for medical personnel to familiarize themselves with medical terms in Spanish in order to improve communication with those who have a limited command of English.

The purpose of this book is to facilitate dialogue between health care professionals and those patients who speak only Spanish. It is divided into several chapters based on presenting chief complaint. Each chapter contains a series of questions that require a simple *yes* or *no* answer. We also included common terms and phrases (which may be used during physical examination and in explaining work up plans, diagnoses, and disposition) and specific discharge instructions for each complaint. Novices, as well as those with some knowledge of Spanish, can easily use this manual by reading the phonetic pronunciation of the Spanish words and phrases.

Physicians, nurses, medical students, paramedics, and medical technicians will find the manual ideal for use in their practice, emergency departments, out-patient clinics, and hospital wards. While it may be used to obtain pertinent information from Spanish-speaking patients, *Medical Spanish: An Instant Translator* should not substitute for the skills and experience of a bilingual health care professional.

Isam Nasr
Marco Cordero

Contents

Part **G**

Miscellaneous   289

Section **III**

Pediatric Chief Complaints   331

Appendix: Pronunciation   379

Index   383

Introduction

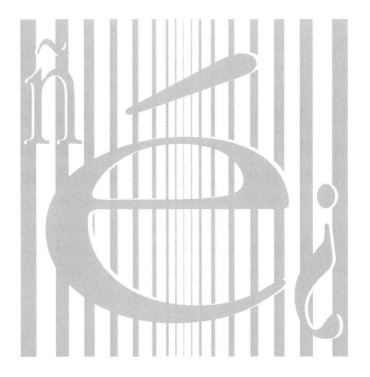

Anatomy	Anatomía	Ah-nah-toh-**mee**-ah
abdomen	el abdomen	ehl ab-**doh**-mehn
ankle	el tobillo	ehl toh-**bee**-yoh
anus	el ano	ehl **ah**-noh
appendix	el apéndice	ehl ah-**pehn**-dee-seh
arm	el brazo	ehl **brah**-soh
artery	la arteria	lah ahr-**teh**-ree-ah
axilla	la axila	lah ak-**see**-lah
back	la espalda	lah ehs-**pahl**-dah
bladder	la vejiga	lah beh-**hee**-gah
body	el cuerpo	ehl **kwehr**-poh
bone	el hueso	ehl **weh**-soh
brain	el cerebro	ehl seh-**reh**-broh
breasts	los senos	lohs **seh**-nohs
buttock	la nalga	la **nahl**-gah
calf	la pantorrilla	lah pahn-toh-**ree**-yhah
cervix	el cuello uterino	ehl **kweh**-yoh oo-teh-**ree**-noh
cheek	la mejilla	lah meh-**hee**-yhah
chest	el pecho	ehl **peh**-choh
chin	el mentón	ehl mehn-**tohn**

clavicle	la clavícula	lah klah-**bee**-kuh-lah
ear (inner / outer)	el oído / la oreja	ehl oh-**ee**-doh / lah oh-**reh**-ha
elbow	el codo	ehl **koh**-doh
eye	el ojo	ehl **oh**-hoh
eyebrow	la ceja	lah **seh**-hah
eyelash	la pestaña	lah pehs-**tah**-nyah
eyelid	el párpado	ehl **pahr**-pah-doh
face	la cara	lah **kah**-rah
finger	el dedo	ehl **deh**-doh
fingernail	la uña	lah **oo**-nyah
foot	el pie	ehl pee-**eh**
forearm	el antebrazo	ehl ahn-teh-**brah**-soh
forehead	la frente	lah **frehn**-teh
gallbladder	la vesícula biliar	lah beh-**see**-koo-lah bee-lee-**ahr**
groin	la ingle	lah **een**-gleh
hair	el pelo / el cabello	ehl **peh**-loh / ehl kah-**beh**-yhoh
hand	la mano	lah **mah**-noh
head	la cabeza	lah kah-**beh**-sah
heart	el corazón	ehl koh-rah-**sohn**
heel	el talón	ehl tah-**lohn**

hip	la cadera	lah kah-**deh**-rah
intestines	los intestinos	lohs een-tehs-**tee**-nohs
joint	la articulación	lah ahr-tee-koo-lah-see-**ohn**
kidney	el riñón	ehl ree-**nyohn**
knee	la rodilla	lah roh-**dee**-yhah
larynx	la laringe	lah lah-**reen**-heh
leg	la pierna	lah pee-**ehr**-nah
lips	los labios	lohs **lah**-bee-ohs
liver	el hígado	ehl **ee**-gah-doh
lung	el pulmón	ehl pool-**mohn**
mandible	la mandíbula	lah mahn-**dee**-boo-lah
mouth	la boca	lah **boh**-kah
muscle	el músculo	ehl **moos**-koo-loh
navel	el ombligo	ehl ohm-**blee**-goh
neck	el cuello	ehl **kweh**-yoh
nerve	el nervio	ehl **nehr**-bee-oh
nipple	el pezón	ehl peh-**sohn**
nose	la nariz	lah nah-**rees**
ovary	el ovario	ehl oh-**bah**-ree-oh
pancreas	el páncreas	ehl **pahn**-kreh-ahs

pelvis	la pelvis	lah **pehl**-bees
penis	el pene	ehl **peh**-neh
prostate	la próstata	lah **prohs**-tah-tah
pupil	la pupila	lah poo-**pee**-lah
rectum	el recto	ehl **rehk**-toh
rib	la costilla	lah kohs-**tee**-yah
scalp	el cuero cabelludo	ehl **kweh**-roh kah-beh-**yuh**-doh
scapula	el ómoplato	ehl **oh**-moh-plah-toh
scrotum	el escroto	ehl ehs-**kroh**-toh
shoulder	el hombro	ehl **ohm**-broh
skin	la piel	lah pee-**ehl**
skull	el cráneo	ehl **krah**-neh-oh
spine	el espinazo	ehl ehs-pee-**nah**-soh
spleen	el bazo	ehl **bah**-soh
sternum	el esternón	ehl ehs-tehr-**nohn**
stomach	el estómago	ehl ehs-**toh**-mah-goh
tendon	el tendón	ehl tehn-**dohn**
testicle	el testículo	ehl tehs-**tee**-koo-loh
thigh	el muslo	ehl **moos**-loh
thorax	el tórax	ehl **toh**-raks
throat	la garganta	lah gahr-**gahn**-tah

thumb	el pulgar	ehl pool-**gahr**
thyroid	la tiroides	lah tee-**roh**-ee-dehs
toes (*on one foot*)	los dedos del pie	lohs **deh**-dohs dehl pee-**eh**
(*on both feet*)	los dedos de los pies	lohs **deh**-dohs deh lohs pee-**ehs**
tongue	la lengua	lah **lehn**-gwah
tonsils	las anginas	lahs ahn-**hee**-nahs
tooth	el diente	ehl dee-**ehn**-teh
trachea	la tráquea	lah **trah**-keh-ah
tubes	los tubos	lohs **too**-bohs
urethra	la uretra	lah oo-**reh**-trah
uterus	el útero / la matriz	ehl **oo**-teh-roh / lah mah-**trees**
uvula	la campanilla	lah kahm-pah-**nee**-yhah
vagina	la vagina	lah bah-**hee**-nah
vein	la vena	lah **beh**-nah
waist	la cintura	lah seen-**too**-rah
wrist	la muñeca	lah moo-**nyeh**-kah

Common Terms

Is there someone with you who speaks English?

¿Hay alguien con usted que hable inglés?
Ah-ee **ahl**-gee-ehn kohn oos-**tehd** keh **ah**-bleh een-**glehs**?

I speak a little Spanish. Please answer *yes* or *no* to the following questions.

Hablo un poco de español. Por favor conteste *sí* o *no* a las siguientes preguntas.
Ah-bloh oon **poh**-koh deh ehs-pah-**nyohl**. Pohr fah-**borh** kohn-**tehs**-teh *see* oh *noh* ah lahs see-gee-**ehn**-tehs preh-**goon**-tahs.

Speak slowly, please.

Hable despacio, por favor.
Ah-bleh dehs-**pah**-see-oh, pohr fah-**bohr**.

Hello.

Hola.
Oh-lah.

Good morning.

Buenos días.
Bweh-nohs **dee**-ahs.

Good afternoon.

Buenas tardes.
Bweh-nahs **tahr**-dehs.

Good evening / night.

Buenas noches.
Bweh-nahs **noh**-chehs.

I am the doctor (*male*).

Soy el doctor.
Soy ehl dohk-**tohr**.

I am the doctor (*female*).

Soy la doctora.
Soy lah dohk-**toh**-rah.

I am the nurse.	Soy la enfermera. Soy lah ehn-fehr-**meh**-rah.
How are you?	¿Cómo está usted? **Koh**-moh ehs-**tah** oos-**tehd**?
How do you feel?	¿Cómo se siente? **Koh**-moh seh see-**ehn**-teh?
What is the problem?	¿Cuál es el problema? **Kwahl ehs** ehl proh-**bleh**-mah?
Have you had this problem before?	¿Ha tenido este problema antes? Ah teh-**nee**-doh **ehs**-teh proh-**bleh**-mah **ahn**-tehs?
Where is your pain?	¿Dónde tiene el dolor? **Dohn**-deh tee-**eh**-neh ehl doh-**lohr**?
Where does it hurt?	¿Dónde le duele? **Dohn**-deh leh **dweh**-leh?
Where does it hurt the most?	¿Dónde le duele más? **Dohn**-deh leh **dweh**-leh mahs?
Show me.	Enséñeme. Ehn-**seh**-nyeh-meh.
When?	¿Cuándo? **Kwahn**-doh?
How?	¿Cómo? **Koh**-moh?
For how long?	¿Por cuánto tiempo? Pohr **kwahn**-toh tee-**ehm**-poh?
Why?	¿Por qué? Pohr **keh**?

Sit down, please.

Siéntese, por favor.
See-**ehn**-teh-seh, pohr fah-**bohr**.

Lie down.

Acuéstese.
Ah-**kwehs**-teh-seh.

Get up.

Levántese.
Leh-**bahn**-teh-seh.

Stand up.

Párese.
Pah-reh-seh.

Turn around.

Voltéese.
Bohl-**teh**-eh-seh.

Turn on your right (left) side.

Voltéese del lado derecho (izquierdo).
Bohl-**teh**-eh-seh dehl **lah**-doh deh-**reh**-choh (ees-kee-**ehr**-doh).

Lie on your back.

Acuéstese boca arriba.
Ah-**kwehs**-teh-seh **boh**-kah ah-**ree**-bah.

Lie on your stomach.

Acuéstese boca abajo.
Ah-**kwehs**-teh-seh **boh**-kah ah-**bah**-hoh.

Relax, please.

Por favor, relájese.
Pohr fah-**bohr**, reh-**lah**-heh-seh.

Calm down.

Cálmese.
Kahl-meh-seh.

Don't move.

No se mueva.
Noh seh **mweh**-bah.

Raise up your head.

Levante la cabeza.
Leh-**bahn**-teh lah kah-**beh**-sah.

Bend over.	Dóblese / Agáchese. **Doh**-bleh-seh / Ah-**gah**-cheh-seh.
Turn your head and cough.	Voltee la cabeza y tosa. Bohl-**teh**-eh lah kah-**beh**-sah ee **toh**-sah.
Take off your clothes.	Quítese la ropa. **Kee**-teh-seh lah **roh**-pah.
Take off your underwear.	Quítese la ropa interior. **Kee**-teh-seh lah **roh**-pah een-teh-ree-**ohr**.
You can get undressed.	Puede desvestirse. **Pweh**-deh dehs-behs-**teer**-seh.
Put on your gown with the open side facing back.	Póngase la bata con la abertura hacia atrás. **Pohn**-gah-seh lah **bah**-tah kohn lah ah-behr-**too**-rah **ah**-see-ah ah-**trahs**.
Put on your clothes.	Póngase la ropa. **Pohn**-gah-seh lah **roh**-pah.
You can get dressed.	Puede vestirse. **Pweh**-deh vehs-**teer**-seh.
You need stitches.	Usted necesita puntadas / suturas. Oos-**tehd** neh-seh-**see**-tah poon-**tah**-dahs / soo-**too**-rahs.
You need an operation.	Usted necesita una operación. Oos-**tehd** neh-seh-**see**-tah **oo**-nah oh-peh-rah-see-**ohn**.
You need an injection.	Usted necesita una inyección. Oos-**tehd** neh-seh-**see**-tah **oo**-nah een-yek-see-**ohn**.

You need to take medicine / medication.	Usted necesita tomar medicina. Oos-**tehd** neh-seh-**see**-tah toh-**mahr** meh-dee-**see**-nah.
You need blood tests.	Usted necesita análisis de sangre. Oos-**tehd** neh-seh-**see**-tah ah-**nah**-lee-sehs deh **sahn**-greh.
You need an X ray.	Usted necesita una radiografía / unos rayos X. Oos-**tehd** neh-seh-**see**-tah **oo**-nah rah-dee oh-grah-**fee**-ah / **oo**-nos **rah**-yohs-**eh**-kees.
You need a cast.	Usted necesita yeso. Oos-**tehd** neh-seh-**see**-tah **yeh**-soh.
You need an ultrasound.	Usted necesita un ultrasonido. Oos-**tehd** neh-seh-**see**-tah oon ool-trah-soh-**nee**-doh.
You need a urine test.	Usted necesita una prueba de orina. Oos-**tehd** neh-seh-**see**-tah **oo**-nah **prweh**-bah deh oh-**ree**-nah.
You need a Foley catheter.	Usted necesita una sonda. Oos-**tehd** neh-seh-**see**-tah **oo**-nah **sohn**-dah.
I need to do a rectal exam.	Necesito hacerle un examen del recto. Neh-seh-**see**-toh ah-**sehr**-leh **oon** ek-**sah**-mehn dehl **rek**-toh.
I need to do a vaginal exam.	Necesito hacerle un examen vaginal. Neh-seh-**see**-toh ah-**sehr**-leh oon ek-**sah**-mehn bah-hee-**nahl**.

I need to examine you for a hernia.	Necesito examinarlo para ver si tiene una hernia. **Neh**-seh-**see**-toh ek-sah-mee-**nahr**-loh **pah**-rah vehr see tee-**eh**-neh **oo**-nah **ehr**-nee-ah.
We are going to give you an IV.	Vamos a ponerle suero intravenoso. **Bah**-mohs ah poh-**nehr**-leh soo-**eh**-roh een-trah-beh-**noh**-soh.
You have an infection.	Usted tiene una infección. Oos-**tehd** tee-**eh**-neh **oo**-nah een-fek-see-**ohn**.
You have diabetes.	Usted tiene diabetes. Oos-**tehd** tee-**eh**-neh dee-ah-**beh**-tehs.
You have a fracture.	Usted tiene una fractura. Oos-**tehd** tee-**eh**-neh **oo**-nah frak-**too**-rah.
You have a sprain.	Usted tiene una torcedura. Oos-**tehd** tee-**eh**-neh **oo**-nah tohr-seh-**doo**-rah.
You have pneumonia.	Usted tiene pulmonía. Oos-**tehd** tee-**eh**-neh pool-moh-**nee**-ah.
You have heart disease.	Usted tiene una enfermedad del corazón. Oos-**tehd** tee-**eh**-neh **oo**-nah ehn-fehr-meh-**dahd** dehl koh-rah-**sohn**.
You have high blood pressure.	Usted tiene alta presión de la sangre. Oos-**tehd** tee-**eh**-neh **ahl**-tah preh-see-**ohn** deh lah **sahn**-greh.

You have low blood pressure.	Usted tiene baja presión de la sangre. Oos-**tehd** tee-**eh**-neh **bah**-ha preh-see-**ohn** deh lah **sahn**-greh.
Take your medicine . . .	Tome su medicina... **Toh**-meh soo meh-dee-**see**-nah...
once a day.	una vez al día. **oo**-nah **behs** ahl **dee**-ah.
twice a day.	dos veces al día. dohs **beh**-sehs ahl **dee**-ah.
three times a day.	tres veces al día. trehs **beh**-sehs ahl **dee**-ah.
four times a day.	cuatro veces al día. **kwah**-troh **beh**-sehs ahl **dee**-ah.
every twelve hours.	cada doce horas. **kah**-dah **doh**-seh **oh**-rahs.
every six hours.	cada seis horas. **kah**-dah **seh**-ees **oh**-rahs.
every eight hours.	cada ocho horas. **kah**-dah **oh**-choh **oh**-rahs.
with food.	con comida. kohn koh-**mee**-dah.
after food / meals.	después de la comida. dehs-**pwehs** deh lah koh-**mee**-dah.
before bed.	antes de acostarse. **ahn**-tehs deh ah-kohs-**tahr**-seh.

before you go to sleep.	antes de dormirse. **ahn**-tehs deh dohr-**meer**-seh.
Avoid alcohol / beer.	Evite el alcohol / la cerveza. Eh-**bee**-teh ehl ahl-**kohl** / lah sehr-**beh**-sah.
Stop taking . . .	Deje de tomar... **Deh**-heh deh toh-**mahr**...
You need to see a specialist.	Usted necesita ver a un especialista. Oos-**tehd** neh-seh-**see**-tah **behr** ah oon ehs-peh-see-ah-**lees**-tah.
You need to return here.	Usted necesita regresar aquí. Oos-**tehd** neh-seh-**see**-tah reh-greh-**sahr** ah-**kee**.
We need to admit you (*male*).	Necesitamos internarlo / admitirlo. Neh-seh-see-**tah**-mohs een-tehr-**nahr**-loh / ahd-mee-**teer**-loh.
We need to admit you (*female*).	Necesitamos internarla / admitirla. Neh-seh-see-**tah**-mohs een-tehr-**nahr**-lah / ahd-mee-**teer**-lah.

Miscellaneous Terms

admit	internar	een-tehr-**nahr**
discharge	dar de alta	**dahr** deh **ahl**-tah
appointment	cita	**see**-tah
blister	ampolla	ahm-**poh**-yah
blood	sangre	**sahn**-greh
blood clot	coágulo de sangre	koh-**ah**-goo-loh deh **sahn**-greh
bruise	moretón	moh-reh-**tohn**
burning	ardor	ahr-**dohr**
capsule	cápsula	**kap**-soo-lah
chills	escalofríos	ehs-kah-loh-**free**-ohs
cramp	calambre	kah-**lahm**-breh
discharge	deshecho	dehs-**eh**-choh
dizziness	mareos	mah-**reh**-ohs
faint	desmayo	dehs-**mah**-yoh
feces	heces	**eh**-sehs
fever	fiebre	fee-**eh**-breh
fracture	fractura	frak-**too**-rah
injection	inyección	een-jeg-see-**ohn**

itch, itching	comezón	koh-meh-**sohn**
lotion	loción	loh-see-**ohn**
mucus	mucosidad	moo-koh-see-**dahd**
ointment	pomada	poh-**mah**-dah
pain	dolor	doh-**lohr**
phlegm	flema	**fleh**-mah
pill	píldora / pastilla	**peel**-doh-rah / pahs-**tee**-yah
rash	salpullido	sahl-poo-**yee**-doh
saliva	saliva	sah-**lee**-bah
sprain	torcedura	tohr-seh-**doo**-rah
sweat	sudor	soo-**dohr**
tablet	tableta	tah-**bleh**-tah
tear	lágrima	**lah**-gree-mah
urine	orina	oh-**ree**-nah
vomit	vómito	**boh**-mee-toh
dizzy	mareado / -a	mah-reh-**ah**-doh / -dah
numb (*adj.*)	entumido / -a	ehn-too-mee-doh / -dah
swollen	hinchado / -a	een-**chah**-doh / -dah

Cardinal Numbers

zero	cero	**seh**-roh
one	uno	**oo**-noh
two	dos	dohs
three	tres	trehs
four	cuatro	**kwah**-troh
five	cinco	**seen**-koh
six	seis	**seh**-ees
seven	siete	see-**eh**-teh
eight	ocho	**oh**-choh
nine	nueve	**nweh**-beh
ten	diez	dee-**ehs**
eleven	once	**ohn**-seh
twelve	doce	**doh**-seh
thirteen	trece	**treh**-seh
fourteen	catorce	kah-**tohr**-seh
fifteen	quince	**keen**-seh
sixteen	dieciséis	dee-eh-see-**say**-ees
seventeen	diecisiete	dee-eh-see-see-**eh**-teh
eighteen	dieciocho	dee-eh-see-**oh**-choh

nineteen	diecinueve	dee-eh-see-**nweh**-beh
twenty	veinte	**beh**-een-teh
twenty-one	veintiuno	beh-een-tee-**oo**-noh
twenty-two	veintidós	beh-een-tee-**dohs**
twenty-three	veintitrés	beh-een-tee-**trehs**
twenty-four	veinticuatro	beh-een-tee-**kwah**-troh
twenty-five	veinticinco	beh-een-tee-**seen**-koh
twenty-six	veintiséis	beh-een-tee-**say**-ees
twenty-seven	veintisiete	beh-een-tee-see-**eh**-teh
twenty-eight	veintiocho	beh-een-tee-**oh**-choh
twenty-nine	veintinueve	beh-een-tee-**nweh**-beh
thirty	treinta	**treh**-een-tah
thirty-one (-two, . . .)	treinta y uno (dos, ...)	**treh**-een-tah ee **oo**-noh (**dohs**, ...)
forty	cuarenta	kwah-**rehn**-tah
forty-one (-two, . . .)	cuarenta y uno (dos, ...)	kwah-**rehn**-tah ee **oo**-noh (**dohs**, ...)
fifty	cincuenta	seen-**kwehn**-tah
sixty	sesenta	seh-**sehn**-tah
seventy	setenta	seh-**tehn**-tah

eighty	ochenta	oh-**chehn**-tah
ninety	noventa	noh-**behn**-tah
one hundred	cien	see-**ehn**
one hundred one (two, . . .)	ciento uno (dos, ...)	see-**ehn**-toh **oo**-noh (**dohs**, ...)

The Days of the Week

Monday	el lunes	ehl **loo**-nehs
Tuesday	el martes	ehl **mahr**-tehs
Wednesday	el miércoles	ehl mee-**ehr**-koh-lehs
Thursday	el jueves	ehl **hweh**-behs
Friday	el viernes	ehl bee-**ehr**-nehs
Saturday	el sábado	ehl **sah**-bah-doh
Sunday	el domingo	ehl doh-**meen**-goh

The Months of the Year

January	enero	eh-**neh**-roh
February	febrero	feh-**breh**-roh
March	marzo	**mahr**-soh
April	abril	ah-**breel**
May	mayo	**mah**-yoh
June	junio	**hoo**-nee-oh

July	julio	**hoo**-lee-oh
August	agosto	ah-**gohs**-toh
September	septiembre	sep-tee-**ehm**-breh
October	octubre	ok-**too**-breh
November	noviembre	noh-bee-**ehm**-breh
December	diciembre	dee-see-**ehm**-breh

Time

today	hoy	**oh**-ee
tomorrow	mañana	mah-**nyah**-nah
the day after tomorrow	pasado mañana	pah-**sah**-doh mah-**nyah**-nah
yesterday	ayer	ah-**yehr**
the day before yesterday	anteayer	ahn-teh-ah-**yehr**
week	la semana	lah seh-**mah**-nah
next week	la próxima semana	lah **prok**-see-mah seh-**mah**-nah
last week	la semana pasada	lah seh-**mah**-nah pah-**sah**-dah
month	el mes	ehl mehs
year	el año	ehl **ah**-nyoh

(*To give a date in Spanish, use* **el** + *a number* + **de** + *the month. For the first day of the month, use* **el primero de** + *month:* **El 14 de julio. El primero de septiembre.**)

Colors

black	negro / -a	**neh**-groh / -grah
blue	azul	ah-**sool**
brown	café	kah-**feh**
gray	gris	grees
green	verde	**behr**-deh
pink	rosa	**roh**-sah
purple	morado / -a	moh-**rah**-doh / -dah
red	rojo / -a	**roh**-hoh / -hah
white	blanco / -a	**blahn**-koh / -kah
yellow	amarillo / -a	ah-mah-**ree**-yoh / -yah

General Patient Information

Información General del Paciente

Een-fohr-mah-see-ohn he-neh-**rahl** dehl pah-see-**ehn**-teh

Do you speak English?

¿Habla usted inglés?
Ah-blah oos-**tehd** een-**glehs**?

Is there someone with you who speaks English?

¿Hay alguien con usted que hable inglés?
Ah-ee **al**-gee-ehn kohn oos-**tehd** keh **ah**-bleh een-**glehs**?

What is your name?	¿Cómo se llama? **Koh**-moh seh **yah**-mah?
	or ¿Cuál es su nombre? Kwahl ehs soo **nohm**-breh?
What is your last name?	¿Cuál es su apellido? Kwahl ehs soo ah-peh-**yee**-doh?
What is your address?	¿Cuál es su dirección? Kwahl ehs soo dee-rek-see-**ohn**?
What is your telephone number?	¿Cuál es su número de teléfono? Kwahl ehs soo **noo**-meh-roh deh teh-**leh**-foh-noh?
How old are you?	¿Cuántos años tiene? **Kwahn**-tohs **ah**-nyohs tee-**eh**-neh?
Are you . . .	¿Es usted... Ehs oos-**tehd**...
married?	casado / -a? kah-**sah**-doh / -dah?
single?	soltero / -a? sol-**teh**-roh / -rah?
widowed?	viudo / -a? vee-**oo**-doh / -dah?
divorced?	divorciado / -a? dee-vohr-see-**ah**-doh / -dah?
separated?	separado / -a? seh-pah-**rah**-doh / -dah?

What is your social security number?	¿Cuál es su número de seguro social? Kwahl ehs soo **noo**-meh-roh deh seh-**goo**-roh soh-see-**ahl**?
In case of emergency whom do you want us to notify?	¿En caso de emergencia, a quien quiere que notifiquemos? Ehn **kah**-soh deh eh-mehr-**hen**-see-ah, ah kee-**ehn** kee-**eh**-reh keh no-tee-fee-**keh**-mos?
What type of insurance do you have?	¿Qué tipo de seguro médico tiene? Keh **tee**-poh deh seh-**goo**-roh **meh**-dee-koh tee-**eh**-neh?
None?	¿Ninguno? Neen-**goo**-noh?
HMO / PPO?	¿HMO / PPO?
Social security?	¿Seguro social? Seh-**goo**-roh soh-see-**ahl**?
Public aid?	¿Ayuda pública? Ah-**yoo**-dah **poo**-blee-kah?
Did you bring your insurance card?	¿Trajo su tarjeta de seguro médico? **Trah**-hoh soo tahr-**heh**-tah deh seh-**goo**-roh **meh**-dee-koh?
What is your doctor's name?	¿Cuál es el nombre de su doctor? Kwahl ehs ehl **nohm**-breh deh soo dohk-**tohr**?
What is your religion?	¿Cuál es su religión? Kwahl ehs soo reh-lee-hee-**ohn**?

Triage Questions

Preguntas de Evaluación
Preh-**goon**-tahs deh eh-vah-loo-ah-see-**ohn**

What is the problem?

¿Cuál es el problema?
Kwahl ehs ehl proh-**bleh**-mah?

When did the problem start?

¿Cuándo empezó el problema?
Kwahn-doh ehm-peh-**soh** ehl proh-**bleh**-mah?

(X) hours ago.

(X) horas.
(X) **oh**-rahs.

(X) days ago.

(X) días.
(X) **dee**-ahs.

(X) months ago.

(X) meses.
(X) **meh**-sehs.

Where do you have the pain?

¿Dónde tiene el dolor?
Dohn-deh tee-**eh**-neh ehl doh-**lohr**?

Do you have a fever?

¿Tiene fiebre?
Tee-**eh**-neh fee-**eh**-breh?

Do you have nausea or vomiting?

¿Tiene náusea o vómito?
Tee-**eh**-neh **nah**-oo-seh-ah oh **boh**-mee-toh?

Do you have any medical problems like . . .

¿Usted tiene algún problema médico como...
Oos-**tehd** tee-**eh**-neh ahl-**goon** proh-**bleh**-mah **meh**-dee-koh **koh**-moh...

high blood pressure?

alta presión de la sangre?
ahl-tah preh-see-**ohn** deh lah **sahn**-greh?

diabetes?	diabetes? dee-ah-**beh**-tehs?
asthma?	asma? **ahs**-mah?
epilepsy?	epilepsia? eh-pee-**lep**-see-ah?
heart disease?	enfermedad del corazón? ehn-fehr-meh-**dad** dehl koh-rah-**sohn**?
stomach ulcers?	úlceras del estomago? **ool**-seh-rahs dehl ehs-**toh**- mah-goh?
Do you take medicine?	¿Toma usted medicina? **Toh**-mah oos-**tehd** meh-dee- **see**-nah?
Did you bring the medicine?	¿Trajo usted la medicina? **Trah**-hoh oos-**tehd** lah meh- dee-**see**-nah?
Did you take anything for . . .	¿Tomó algo para... Toh-**moh ahl**-goh **pah**-rah...
the pain?	el dolor? ehl doh-**lohr**?
the fever?	la fiebre? lah fee-**eh**-breh?
the vomiting?	el vómito? ehl **boh**-mee-toh?
What did you take?	¿Qué tomó? Keh toh-**moh**?

(*For a woman*) When was your last period?	¿Cuándo fue su última regla / período? **Kwahn**-doh fweh soo **ool**-tee-mah **reh**-glah / peh-**ree**-oh-doh?
Are you allergic to . . .	¿Es usted alérgico / a a... Ehs oos-**tehd** ah-**lehr**-hee-koh / -kah a...
penicillin?	penicilina? peh-nee-see-**lee**-nah?
sulfa?	sulfa? **sool**-fah?
iodine?	iodo? **yoh**-doh?
aspirin?	aspirina? ahs-pee-**ree**-nah?
shrimp?	camarones? kah-mah-**roh**-nehs?
peanuts?	cacahuates? kah-kah-**hwah**-tehs?
When was the last time you received a tetanus vaccine?	¿Cuándo fue la última vez que recibió una vacuna del tétano? **Kwahn**-doh fweh lah **ool**-tee-mah vehs keh reh-see-bee-**oh** **oo**-nah vah-**koo**-nah dehl **teh**-tah-noh?
How much do you weigh?	¿Cuánto pesa usted? **Kwahn**-toh **peh**-sah oos-**tehd**?
How tall are you?	¿Cuánto mide de altura? **Kwahn**-toh **mee**-deh deh ahl-**too**-rah?

Pain

Dolor
Doh-**lohr**

Where do you have the pain?

¿Dónde tiene el dolor?
Dohn-deh tee-**eh**-neh ehl doh-**lohr**?

When did the pain start?

¿Cuándo empezó el dolor?
Kwahn-doh ehm-peh-**soh** ehl doh-**lohr**?

Where did the pain start?

¿Dónde empezó el dolor?
Dohn-deh ehm-peh-**soh** ehl doh-**lohr**?

Does the pain travel to another place?

¿Le viaja el dolor a otro lugar?
Leh vee-**ah**-hah ehl doh-**lohr** ah **oh**-troh loo-**gahr**?

Point to where the pain travels.

Apunte a dónde le viaja el dolor.
Ah-**poon**-teh ah **dohn**-deh leh bee-**ah**-hah ehl doh-**lohr**.

Does the pain come and go?

¿El dolor le va y viene?
Ehl doh-**lohr** leh bah ee bee-**eh**-neh?

Is the pain constant?

¿Es el dolor constante?
Ehs ehl doh-**lohr** kohns-**tahn**-teh?

How long does the pain last?

¿Cuánto tiempo le dura el dolor?
Kwahn-toh tee-**ehm**-poh leh **doo**-rah ehl doh-**lohr**?

(X) seconds.

(X) segundos.
(X) seh-**goon**-dohs.

(X) minutes.	(X) minutos. (X) mee-**noo**-tohs.
(X) hours.	(X) horas. (X) **oh**-rahs.
What is the pain like?	¿Cómo es el dolor? **Koh**-moh ehs ehl doh-**lohr**?
Is it acute / sharp?	¿Es agudo? Ehs ah-**goo**-doh?
Is it severe?	¿Es severo? Ehs seh-**beh**-roh?
Is it like a knife?	¿Es como cuchillo? Ehs **koh**-moh koo-**chee**-yoh?
Does it ache?	¿Es adolorido? Ehs ah-doh-loh-**ree**-doh?
Does it burn?	¿Es quemante? Ehs keh-**mahn**-teh?
Is it like a pressure?	¿Es opresivo? Ehs oh-preh-**see**-boh?
Is it like cramps?	¿Es como calambres? Ehs **koh**-moh kah-**lahm**-brehs?
Have you had this type of pain before?	¿Ha tenido este tipo de dolor antes? Ah teh-**nee**-doh **ehs**-teh **tee**-poh deh doh-**lohr ahn**-tehs?
What things cause the pain?	¿Qué cosas le causan el dolor? Keh **koh**-sahs leh **kah**-oo-sahn ehl doh-**lohr**?

What makes the pain better?	¿Qué le mejora el dolor? Keh leh meh-**hoh**-rah ehl doh-**lohr**?
Is the pain the same since it started?	¿Es el dolor igual desde que empezó? Ehs ehl doh-**lohr** ee-**gwahl dehs**-deh keh ehm-peh-**soh**?
better	mejor meh-**hohr**
worse	peor peh-**ohr**
Have you taken something for the pain?	¿Ha tomado algo para el dolor? Ah toh-**mah**-doh **ahl**-goh **pah**-rah ehl doh-**lohr**?
Tylenol?	¿Tylenol? **Tay**-leh-nohl?
Aspirin?	¿Aspirinas? Ahs-pee-**ree**-nahs?
Ibuprofen?	¿Ibuprofen? Ee-boo-**proh**-fehn?
Alcohol?	¿bebidas alcohólicas? beh-**bee**-dahs ahl-**koh**-lee-kahs?
Something else?	¿Otra cosa? **Oh**-trah **koh**-sah?

Adult Chief Complaints

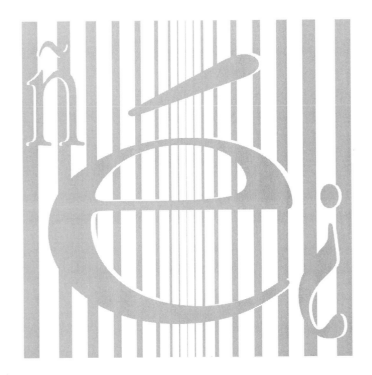

Head and Neck

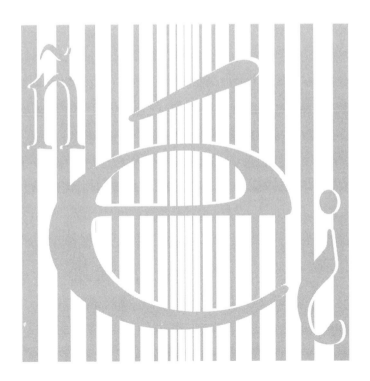

Sore Throat

Dolor de Garganta
Doh-**lohr** deh gahr-**gahn**-tah

Do you have pain in your throat?

¿Tiene dolor en la garganta?
Tee-**eh**-neh doh-**lohr** ehn lah gahr-**gahn**-tah?

How many days have you had the pain?

¿Por cuántos días ha tenido el dolor?
Pohr **kwahn**-tohs **dee**-ahs ah teh-**nee**-doh ehl doh-**lohr**?

Do you have pain when you swallow?

¿Tiene dolor para pasar saliva o al tragar?
Tee-**eh**-neh doh-**lohr pah**-rah pah-**sahr** sah-**lee**-bah o ahl trah-**gahr**?

Can you drink fluids?

¿Puede tomar líquidos?
Pweh-deh toh-**mahr lee**-kee-dohs?

Have you noticed a change in your voice?

¿Ha notado cambio en su voz?
Ah noh-**tah**-doh **kahm**-bee-oh ehn soo bohs?

Are you hoarse?

¿Está ronco / a?
Ehs-**tah rohn**-koh / -kah?

Are you drooling?

¿Babea?
Bah-**beh**-ah?

Do you have a fever?

¿Tiene fiebre?
Tee-**eh**-neh fee-**eh**-breh?

Do you have trouble breathing?

¿Tiene problemas al respirar?
Tee-**eh**-neh proh-**bleh**-mahs ahl rehs-pee-**rahr**?

Do you have a cough?	¿Tiene tos? Tee-**eh**-neh tohs?
Do you have an earache?	¿Tiene dolor de oído? Tee-**eh**-neh doh-**lohr** deh oh-**ee**-doh?
Do you have a headache?	¿Tiene dolor de cabeza? Tee-**eh**-neh doh-**lohr** deh kah-**beh**-sah?
Do you have abdominal pain?	¿Tiene dolor en el abdomen? Tee-**eh**-neh doh-**lohr** ehn ehl ab-**doh**-mehn?
Have you had vomiting?	¿Ha tenido vómito? Ah teh-**nee**-doh **boh**-mee-toh?
Have you had throat infections before?	¿Ha tenido infecciones en la garganta antes? Ah teh-**nee**-doh een-fek-see-**ohn**-ehs ehn lah gahr-**gahn**-tah **ahn**-tehs?
Have you (recently) been in contact with a person with a sore throat?	¿Ha estado en contacto (recientemente) con una persona a quien le duela la garganta? Ah ehs-**tah**-doh ehn kohn-**tak**-toh (reh-see-**ehn**-teh-**mehn**-teh) kohn **oo**-nah pehr-**soh**-nah ah kee-**ehn** leh **dweh**-lah lah gahr-**gahn**-tah?
Do you smoke?	¿Fuma usted? **Foo**-mah oos-**tehd**?
How many cigarettes do you smoke a day?	¿Cuántos cigarrillos fuma usted por día? **Kwahn**-tohs see-gah-**ree**-yohs **foo**-mah oos-**tehd** pohr **dee**-ah?

Do you have a rash?

¿Tiene manchas / ronchas en
la piel?
Tee-**eh**-neh **mahn**-chahs / **rohn**-
chahs ehn lah pee-**ehl**?

Do you have allergies?

¿Tiene alergias?
Tee-**eh**-neh ah-**lehr**-hee-ahs?

Are you allergic to
penicillin?

¿Es alérgico / a la
penicilina?
Ehs-ah-**lehr**-hee-koh / -kah
lah peh-nee-see-**lee**-nah?

Common Phrases for the Exam for the Sore Throat

Open your mouth.

Abra la boca.
Ah-brah lah **boh**-kah.

Stick out your tongue.

Saque la lengua.
Sah-keh lah **lehn**-gwah.

Say "aah."

Diga "aah."
Dee-gah "aaahhh."

I need to do a throat culture.

Necesito hacerle un cultivo de
garganta.
Neh-seh-**see**-toh ah-**sehr**-leh
oon kool-**tee**-boh deh gahr-
gahn-tah.

You have a throat infection.

Usted tiene una infección de
la garganta.
Oos-**tehd** tee-**eh**-neh **oo**-nah
een-fek-see-**ohn** deh lah gahr-
gahn-tah.

You have an abscess in your
tonsil.

Usted tiene un absceso en la
amígdala.
Oos-**tehd** tee-**eh**-neh oon ahb-
seh-soh ehn lah ah-**meeg**-dah-
lah.

I am going to give you an injection.	Le voy a dar una inyección. Leh boy ah dahr **oo**-nah een-yek-see-**ohn**.
I am going to give you pills (antibiotics) for the infection.	Le voy a dar pastillas (antibióticos) para la infección. Leh boy ah dahr pahs-**tee**-yahs (ahn-tee-bee-**oh**-tee-kohs) **pah**-rah lah een-fek-see-**ohn**.

Discharge Instructions for Sore Throat

See your doctor if . . .	Vea a su médico si... **Beh**-ah ah soo **meh**-dee-koh see...
you have trouble breathing,	tiene dificultad para respirar, tee-**eh**-neh dee-fee-kool-**tahd pah**-rah rehs-pee-**rahr**,
you have trouble swallowing,	tiene dificultad para tragar, tee-**eh**-neh dee-fee-kool-**tahd pah**-rah trah-**gahr**,
the fever doesn't go away in two days,	no se le quita la fiebre en dos días, noh seh leh **kee**-tah lah fee-**eh**-breh ehn dohs **dee**-ahs,
you are not feeling better.	no se siente mejor. noh seh see-**ehn**-teh meh-**hor**.
Take two Tylenol tablets every four to six hours as needed for fever.	Tome dos tabletas de Tylenol cada cuatro a seis horas si es necesario para la fiebre. **Toh**-meh dohs tah-**bleh**-tahs

deh **Tay**-leh-nohl **kah**-dah
kwah-troh ah **seh**-ees **oh**-rahs
see ehs neh-seh-**sah**-ree-oh
pah-rah lah fee-**eh**-breh.

Take one tablet of the
antibiotic (penicillin) every six
hours.

Tome una tableta del
antibiótico (de la penicilina)
cada seis horas.
Toh-meh **ooh**-nah tah-**bleh**-tah
dehl ahn-tee-bee-**oh**-tee-koh
(deh lah peh-nee-see-**lee**-nah)
kah-dah **seh**-ees **oh**-rahs.

Red Eye

Ojo Rojo

Oh-hoh **roh**-ho

Do you have pain in the eye?

¿Tiene dolor en el ojo?
Tee-**eh**-neh doh-**lohr** ehn ehl
oh-hoh?

Since when has it been red?

¿Desde cuándo lo tiene rojo?
Dehs-deh **kwahn**-doh loh tee-
eh-neh **roh**-ho?

Today only?

¿Hoy solamente?
Oy soh-lah-**mehn**-teh?

How many days?

¿Cuántos días?
Kwahn-tohs **dee**-ahs?

Were you hit in the eye?

¿Se pegó en el ojo?
Seh peh-**goh** ehn ehl **oh**-hoh?

Did you get dust in your eye?

¿Le entró polvo en el ojo?
Leh ehn-**troh** **pohl**-boh ehn ehl
oh-hoh?

Where?

¿Dónde?
Dohn-deh?

In the house?	¿En la casa? Ehn lah **kah**-sah?
At work?	¿En el trabajo? Ehn ehl trah-**bah**-ho?
In the street?	¿En la calle? Ehn la **kah**-yeh?
Did you splash household cleaner in your eye?	¿Se salpicó con limpiador de casa en el ojo? Seh sahl-pee-**koh** kohn leem-pee-ah-**dohr** deh **kah**-sah ehn ehl **oh**-hoh?
Did anyone stick his finger in your eye?	¿Alguién le picó el ojo con un dedo? **Ahl**-gee-ehn leh pee-**koh** ehl **oh**-ho kohn oon **deh**-doh?
Do you have a runny eye discharge?	¿Tiene deshecho del ojo? Tee-**eh**-neh dehs-**eh**-choh dehl **oh**-hoh?
What color is it?	¿De qué color es? Deh **keh** koh-**lohr** ehs?
Is it clear?	¿Es claro? Ehs **klah**-roh?
Is it yellow?	¿Es amarillo? Ehs ah-mah-**ree**-yoh?
Is it green?	¿Es verde? Ehs **behr**-deh?
Do you wake up in the morning with your eyes glued shut?	¿Se despierta en la mañana con los ojos cerrados por el deshecho? Seh dehs-pee-**ehr**-tah ehn lah mah-**nyah**-nah kohn lohs **oh**-hohs seh-**rah**-dohs pohr ehl dehs-**eh**-choh?

Do your eyes tear?

¿Le lloran los ojos?
Leh **yoh**-rahn lohs **oh**-hohs?

Do your eyes itch?

¿Le da comezón en los ojos?
Leh dah koh-meh-**sohn** ehn
lohs **oh**-hohs?

Do your eyes burn?

¿Le arden los ojos?
Leh **ahr**-dehn lohs **oh**-hohs?

Does the light bother your eyes?

¿A sus ojos les molesta la luz?
Ah soos **oh**-hohs lehs moh-
lehs-tah lah loos?

Is your vision blurred?

¿Tiene la vista borrosa o nublada?
Tee-**eh**-neh lah **bees**-tah boh-
roh-sah oh noo-**blah**-dah?

Do you see double?

¿Ve usted doble?
Beh oos-**tehd doh**-bleh?

Do you have a headache?

¿Tiene dolor de cabeza?
Tee-**eh**-neh doh-**lohr** deh kah-
beh-sah?

Do you have pain around your eye?

¿Tiene dolor alrededor del ojo?
Tee-**eh**-neh doh-**lohr** ahl-reh-
deh-**dohr** dehl **oh**-hoh?

Do you feel like there is something in your eye?

¿Siente usted como si tuviera algo en el ojo?
See-**ehn**-teh oos-**tehd koh**-moh
see too-bee-**eh**-rah **ahl**-goh
ehn ehl **oh**-hoh?

Do you feel like there is something under your eyelid?

¿Siente como si tuviera algo debajo del párpado?
See-**ehn**-teh **koh**-moh see too-
bee-**eh**-rah **ahl**-goh deh-**bah**-
hoh dehl **par**-pah-doh?

Did you put medicine in your eye?	¿Se puso medicina en el ojo? Seh **poo**-soh meh-dee-**see**-nah ehn ehl **oh**-hoh?
Did you use eye drops?	¿Se puso gotas para los ojos? Seh **poo**-soh **goh**-tahs **pah**-rah lohs **oh**-hohs?
Did you use eye ointment?	¿Se puso pomada para los ojos? Seh **poo**-soh poh-**mah**-dah **pah**-rah lohs **oh**-hohs?
Do you use contact lenses?	¿Usa lentes de contacto? **Oo**-sah **lehn**-tehs deh kohn-**tahk**-toh?
Are they soft or hard contact lenses?	¿Son lentes de contacto suaves o duros? Sohn **lehn**-tehs deh kohn-**tahk**-toh soo-**ah**-behs oh **doo**-rohs?
Did you remove them?	¿Se los quitó? Seh lohs kee-**toh**?
When did you last use them?	¿Cuándo fue la última vez que los usó? **Kwahn**-doh fweh lah **ool**-tee-mah behs keh lohs oo-**soh**?
(X) hours (days) ago.	(X) horas (días). (X) **oh**-rahs (**dee**-ahs).
Do you use prescription eye glasses?	¿Usa usted lentes de aumento? **Oo**-sah oos-**tehd lehn**-tehs deh ah-oo-**mehn**-toh?

Do you know if you have glaucoma?

¿Sabe usted si tiene glaucoma (alta presión dentro del ojo)? Sah-beh oos-**tehd** see tee-**eh**-neh glah-oo-**koh**-mah (**ahl**-tah preh-see-**ohn dehn**-troh dehl **oh**-hoh)?

Do you suffer from high blood pressure?

¿Padece usted de alta presión? Pah-**deh**-seh oos-**tehd** deh **ahl**-tah preh-see-**ohn**?

Do you have cataracts?

¿Tiene usted cataratas? Tee-**eh**-neh oos-**tehd** kah-tah-**rah**-tahs?

Common Phrases for the Exam for Red Eye

Look at the light, please.

Mire la luz, por favor. **Mee**-reh lah loos, pohr fah-**bohr**.

Follow my fingers with your eyes without moving your head.

Siga mis dedos con sus ojos sin mover la cabeza. **See**-gah mees **deh**-dohs kohn soos **oh**-hohs seen moh-**behr** lah kah-**beh**-sah.

Don't move your eyes.

No mueva los ojos. Noh **mweh**-bah lohs **oh**-hohs.

I am going to put in some anesthetic eye drops.

Voy a ponerle a los ojos unas gotas con anestesia. **Boh**-ee ah poh-**nehr**-leh ah lohs **oh**-hohs **oo**-nahs **goh**-tahs kohn ah-nehs-**teh**-see-ah.

You have a bacterial (viral) infection in your eyes.

Tiene una infección bacterial (viral) en los ojos. Tee-**eh**-neh **oo**-nah een-fek-see-**ohn** bahk-teh-ree-**ahl** (bee-**rahl**) ehn lohs **oh**-hohs.

You have glaucoma.	Tiene glaucoma.
	Tee-**eh**-neh glah-oo-**koh**-mah.
You have a piece of metal (wood) in your eye.	Tiene un pedazo de metal (madera) en el ojo.
	Tee-**eh**-neh oon peh-**dah**-soh deh meh-**tahl** (mah-**deh**-rah) ehn ehl **oh**-hoh.
You have a corneal abrasion.	Tiene una raspadura (un rasguño) en la córnea.
	Tee-**eh**-neh **oo**-nah rahs-pah-**doo**-rah (oon rahs-**goo**-nyoh) ehn lah **kohr**-neh-ah.
We are going to put ointment in your eye and patch it.	Vamos a ponerle una pomada en el ojo y cubrirle el ojo con un parche.
	Bah-mohs ah poh-**nehr**-leh **oo**-nah poh-**mah**-dah ehn ehl **oh**-hoh ee koo-**breer**-leh ehl **oh**-ho kohn oon **pahr**-cheh.
Don't take the patch off until you see the eye specialist.	No se quite el parche hasta que lo vea el especialista de los ojos.
	No seh **kee**-teh ehl **pahr**-cheh **ahs**-tah keh loh **be**-ah ehl ehs-peh-see-ah-**lees**-tah deh lohs **oh**-hohs.

Discharge Instructions for Red Eye

Return to the hospital (clinic) if . . .	Regrese al hospital (a la clínica) si...
	Reh-**greh**-seh ahl **ohs**-pee-tahl (ah lah **klee**-nee-kah) see...
you have blurred vision,	tiene la vista borrosa,
	tee-**eh**-neh lah **bees**-tah boh-**roh**-sah,

there is severe pain in the eye,	hay dolor muy fuerte en el ojo, ay doh-**lohr** mooy **fwehr**-teh ehn ehl **oh**-hoh,
or you are not better in two days.	o no se siente mejor en dos días. oh noh seh see-**ehn**-teh meh-**hor** ehn dohs **dee**-ahs.
Come back immediately if it gets worse.	Regrese inmediatamente si se siente peor. Reh-**greh**-seh ee-meh-dee-ah-tah-**mehn**-teh see seh see-**ehn**-teh peh-**ohr**.

Wash your hands after applying the medicine.

Lávese las manos después de ponerse la medicina.
Lah-beh-seh lahs **mah**-nohs dehs-**pwehs** deh poh-**nehr**-seh lah meh-dee-**see**-nah.

Use (X) drops of the medication (Y) times a day.

Use (X) gotas de la medicina (Y) veces al día.
Oo-seh (X) **goh**-tahs deh lah meh-dee-**see**-nah (Y) **beh**-sehs ahl **dee**-ah.

See your doctor on (*date*).

Vea a su médico el (X) de (*month*).
Beh-ah ah soo **meh**-dee-koh ehl (X) deh (*month*).

Earache

Dolor del Oído

Doh-**lohr** dehl oh-**ee**-doh

Do you have pain in your right (left) ear?

¿Tiene dolor en el oído derecho (izquierdo)?
Tee-**eh**-neh doh-**lohr** en ehl oh-**ee**-doh deh-**reh**-choh (ees-kee-**ehr**-doh)?

When did the pain start?

¿Cuándo empezó el dolor?
Kwahn-doh ehm-peh-**soh** ehl doh-**lohr**?

(X) hours ago.

(X) horas.
(X) **oh**-rahs.

(X) days ago.

(X) días.
(X) **dee**-ahs.

(X) weeks ago.

(X) semanas.
(X) seh-**mah**-nahs.

Have you noticed drainage from your ear?

¿Ha notado usted deshecho de su oído?
Ah noh-**tah**-doh oos-**tehd** dehs-**eh**-choh deh soo oh-**ee**-doh?

What color is the drainage?

¿De qué color es el deshecho?
Deh **keh** koh-**lohr** ehs ehl dehs-**eh**-choh?

Is it yellow?

¿Es amarillo?
Ehs ah-mah-**ree**-yoh?

Is it green?

¿Es verde?
Ehs **behr**-deh?

Is it clear?

¿Es claro?
Ehs **klah**-roh?

Do you have wax in your ear?	¿Tiene cerilla en el oído? Tee-**eh**-neh seh-**ree**-yah ehn ehl oh-**ee**-doh?
Do you hear less?	¿Oye usted menos? **Oh**-yeh oos-**tehd meh**-nohs?
Do you have ringing in your ear?	¿Tiene usted zumbido en el oído? Tee-**eh**-neh oos-**tehd** soom-**bee**-doh ehn ehl oh-**ee**-doh?
Did someone hit you in the ear?	¿Le pegó alguien en el oído? Leh peh-**goh ahl**-gee-ehn ehn ehl oh-**ee**-doh?
Did you put something / Did something get in your ear?	¿Se metió algo en el oído? Seh meh-tee-**oh ahl**-goh ehn ehl oh-**ee**-doh?
A Q-tip?	¿Un Q-tip? Oon kee-**uh** teep?
A bobby pin?	¿Un pasador? Oon pah-sah-**dohr**?
An insect?	¿Un insecto? Oon een-**sehk**-toh?
Do you have blood coming from your ear?	¿Le sale sangre del oído? Leh **sah**-leh **sahn**-greh dehl oh-**ee**-doh?
Do you feel something moving in your ear?	¿Siente que algo se mueve dentro de su oído? See-**ehn**-teh keh **ahl**-goh seh **mweh**-beh **dehn**-troh deh soo oh-**ee**-doh?
Do you have fever?	¿Tiene usted fiebre? Tee-**eh**-neh oos-**tehd** fee-**eh**-breh?

Have you had a cold?	¿Ha tenido catarro?
	Ah teh-**nee**-doh kah-**tah**-roh?
Have you had a sore throat?	¿Ha tenido dolor de garganta?
	Ah teh-**nee**-doh doh-**lohr** deh
	gahr-**gahn**-tah?
Have you had ear infections?	¿Ha tenido infecciones del
	oído?
	Ah teh-**nee**-doh een-fek-see-
	ohn-ehs dehl oh-**ee**-doh?
Have you used ear drops?	¿Ha usado gotas para el oído?
	Ah oo-**sah**-doh **goh**-tahs **pah**-
	rah ehl oh-**ee**-doh?
Do you have diabetes?	¿Tiene usted diabetes?
	Tee-**eh**-neh oos-**tehd** dee-ah-
	beh-tehs?
Are you allergic to penicillin?	¿Es alérgico / -a a la penicilina?
	Ehs ah-**lehr**-hee-koh / -kah ah
	lah peh-nee-see-**lee**-nah?

Common Phrases for the Exam for Earache

You have a lot of wax in your ear.	Usted tiene mucha cerilla en el oído.
	Oos-**tehd** tee-**eh**-neh **moo**-chah
	seh-**ree**-yah ehn ehl oh-**ee**-doh.
You have an ear infection.	Usted tiene una infección en el oído.
	Oos-**tehd** tee-**eh**-neh **oo**-nah
	een-fek-see-**ohn** ehn ehl oh-**ee**-
	doh.
You have an infection in the ear canal.	Usted tiene una infección en el canal del oído.
	Oos-**tehd** tee-**eh**-neh **oo**-nah
	een-fek-see-**ohn** ehn ehl kah-
	nahl dehl oh-**ee**-doh.

You have a ruptured tympanic membrane.	Se le rompió la membrana timpánica. Seh leh rohm-pee-**oh** lah mehm-**brah**-nah teem-**pah**-nee-kah.

Discharge Instructions for Earache

Return to the hospital (clinic) if . . .	Regrese al hospital (a la clínica) si... Reh-**greh**-seh ahl ohs-pee-**tahl** (ah lah **klee**-nee-kah) see...
the ear pain gets worse,	el dolor del oído es peor, ehl doh-**lohr** dehl oh-**ee**-doh ehs peh-**ohr**,
you have fever or vomiting,	tiene fiebre o vómito, tee-**eh**-neh fee-**eh**-breh oh **boh**-mee-toh,
you have a headache or a stiff neck,	tiene dolor de cabeza o el cuello tieso, tee-**eh**-neh doh-**lohr** deh kah-**beh**-sah o ehl **kweh**-yoh tee-**eh**-soh,
or you are not better in two days.	o no está mejor en dos días. oh noh ehs-**tah** meh-**hor** ehn dohs **dee**-ahs.
Put two drops in your ear every six hours.	Ponga dos gotas en su oído cada seis horas. **Pohn**-gah dohs **goh**-tahs ehn soo oh-**ee**-doh **kah**-dah **seh**-ees **oh**-rahs.
Take (X) pills every (Y) hours.	Tome (X) pastillas cada (Y) horas. **Toh**-meh (X) pahs-**tee**-yahs **kah**-dah (Y) **oh**-rahs.

Dental Pain

Dolor Dental

Doh-**lohr** dehn-**tahl**

How long have you had the pain?

¿Cuánto tiempo lleva con el dolor?
Kwahn-toh tee-**ehm**-poh **yeh**-bah kohn ehl doh-**lohr**?

Have you seen the dentist?

¿Ha visto al dentista?
Ah **bees**-toh ahl dehn-**tees**-tah?

Show me which tooth hurts.

Enséñeme cuál diente le duele.
Ehn-**seh**-nyeh-meh kwahl dee-**ehn**-teh leh **dweh**-leh.

Have you had trouble with this tooth before?

¿Ha tenido problemas con este diente antes?
Ah tee-**nee**-doh proh-**bleh**-mahs kohn **ehs**-teh dee-**ehn**-teh **ahn**-tehs?

Did you hit your tooth?

¿Se pegó en el diente?
Seh peh-**goh** ehn ehl dee-**ehn**-teh?

Did you bite something hard?

¿Mordió algo duro?
Mohr-dee-**oh** **ahl**-goh **doo**-roh?

Do you know if you have any cavities?

¿Sabe si tiene caries?
Sah-beh see tee-**eh**-neh **kah**-ree-ehs?

Are your gums swollen?

¿Tiene hinchadas las encías?
Tee-**eh**-neh een-**chah**-dahs lahs ehn-**see**-ahs?

Are your gums bleeding?

¿Tiene sangrado de las encías?
Tee-**eh**-neh sahn-**grah**-doh deh lahs ehn-**see**-ahs?

Do you have pus in your gums?

¿Tiene pus en las encías?
Tee-**eh**-neh poos ehn lahs ehn-**see**-ahs?

Is your mandible swollen?

¿Tiene hinchada la mandíbula?
Tee-**eh**-neh een-**chah**-dah lah mahn-**dee**-boo-lah?

Do you have a fever?

¿Tiene fiebre?
Tee-**eh**-neh fee-**eh**-breh?

Do you have swollen lymph nodes in your neck?

¿Tiene hinchados los ganglios linfáticos del cuello?
Tee-**eh**-neh een-**chah**-dohs lohs **gahn**-glee-ohs leen-**fah**-tee-kohs dehl **kweh**-yoh?

What are you taking for the pain?

¿Qué está tomando para el dolor?
Keh ehs-**tah** toh-**mahn**-doh **pah**-rah ehl doh-**lohr**?

Do you have allergies?

¿Tiene alergias?
Tee-**eh**-neh ah-**lehr**-hee-ahs?

Common Phrases for the Exam for Dental Pain

Open your mouth, please.

Abra la boca, por favor.
Ah-brah lah **boh**-kah, pohr fah-**bohr**.

Tell me if it hurts when I touch your tooth.

Dígame si le duele cuando le toco el diente.
Dee-gah-meh see leh **dweh**-leh **kwahn**-doh leh **toh**-koh ehl dee-**ehn**-teh.

I need to get an X-ray of your teeth.

Necesito sacarle una radiografía de los dientes.
Neh-seh-**see**-toh sah-**kahr**-leh **oo**-nah rah-dee-oh-grah-**fee**-ah deh lohs dee-**ehn**-tehs.

You have an abscess in your tooth.	Usted tiene un absceso en un diente.
	Oos-**tehd** tee-**eh**-neh oon ahb-**seh**-soh ehn oon dee-**ehn**-teh.
I am going to give you something for the pain.	Le voy a dar algo para el dolor.
	Leh boy ah dahr **ahl**-goh **pah**-rah ehl doh-**lohr**.
I am going to give you an antibiotic.	Le voy a dar un antibiótico.
	Leh boy ah dahr oon ahn-tee-bee-**oh**-tee-koh.
I am going to anesthetize the tooth.	Le voy a poner anestesia en el diente.
	Leh boy ah poh-**nehr** ah-nehs-**teh**-see-ah ehn ehl dee-**ehn**-teh.
You have an infection of the gums.	Usted tiene una infección de las encías.
	Oos-**tehd** tee-**eh**-neh **oo**-nah een-fek-see-**ohn** deh lahs ehn-**see**-ahs.

Discharge Instructions for Dental Pain

Take your medicine as indicated.	Tome su medicina como le indicaron.
	Toh-meh soo meh-dee-**see**-nah **koh**-moh leh een-dee-**kah**-rohn.
Avoid cold or hot drinks.	Evite bebidas frías o calientes.
	Eh-**bee**-teh beh-**bee**-dahs **free**-ahs oh kah-lee-**ehn**-tehs.
Avoid chewing hard foods.	Evite masticar comidas duras.
	Eh-**bee**-teh mahs-tee-**kahr** koh-**mee**-dahs **doo**-rahs.

You need to see a dentist tomorrow.

Usted necesita ver a un dentista mañana.
Oos-**tehd** neh-seh-**see**-tah behr ah oon dehn-**tees**-tah mah-**nyah**-nah.

Epistaxis

Sangrado Nasal

Sahn-**grah**-doh nah-**sahl**

When did the bleeding start?

¿Cuándo empezó el sangrado?
Kwahn-doh ehm-peh-**soh** ehl sahn-**grah**-doh?

From which side of your nose are you bleeding?

¿De qué lado de la nariz está sangrando?
Deh keh **lah**-doh deh lah nah-**rees** ehs-**tah** sahn-**grahn**-doh?

Did the bleeding start spontaneously?

¿Empezó el sangrado espontáneamente?
Ehm-peh-**soh** ehl sahn-**grah**-doh ehs-pohn-**tah**-neh-ah-mehn-teh?

Have you had bleeding before?

¿Ha tenido sangrado antes?
Ah teh-**nee**-doh sahn-**grah**-doh **ahn**-tehs?

Did someone hit you?

¿Alguien le pegó?
Ahl-gee-ehn leh peh-**goh**?

Did you fall?

¿Se cayó?
Seh kah-**yoh**?

Did you hit yourself against something?

¿Se pegó con algo?
Seh peh-**goh** kohn **ahl**-goh?

Did you put something in your nose?	¿Se metió algo dentro de la nariz? Seh meh-tee-**oh ahl**-goh **dehn**-troh deh lah nah-**rees**?
How long did the bleeding last?	¿Cuánto tiempo duró el sangrado? **Kwahn**-toh tee-**ehm**-poh doo-**roh** ehl sahn-**grah**-doh?
(X) minute.	(X) minutos. (X) mee-**noo**-tohs.
(X) hour.	(X) horas. (X) **oh**-rahs.
How do you stop the bleeding?	¿Cómo para el sangrado? **Koh**-moh **pah**-rah ehl sahn-**grah**-doh?
Do you put a wet rag on your forehead?	¿Pone un trapo húmedo en la frente? **Poh**-neh oon **trah**-poh **oo**-meh-doh ehn lah **frehn**-teh?
Do you put Kleenex or toilet paper in your nostrils?	¿Pone kleenex o papel higiénico en las narices? **Poh**-neh **klee**-neks oh pah-**pehl** ee-hee-**eh**-nee-koh ehn lahs nah-**ree**-sehs?
Do you pinch your nose for a few minutes?	¿Se aprieta la nariz por algunos minutos? Seh ah-pree-**eh**-tah lah nah-**rees** pohr ahl-**goo**-nohs mee-**noo**-tohs?
Do you put your head back?	¿Hace la cabeza hacia atrás? **Ah**-seh lah kah-**beh**-sah **ah**-see-ah ah-**trahs**?

Have you had a cold in the last few days?

¿Ha tenido catarro los últimos días?
Ah teh-**nee**-doh kah-**tah**-roh lohs **ool**-tee-mohs **dee**-ahs?

Do you have high blood pressure?

¿Tiene alta presión de la sangre?
Tee-**eh**-neh **ahl**-tah preh-see-**ohn** deh lah **sahn**-greh?

Do you take medication for high blood pressure?

¿Toma medicina para la alta presión?
Toh-mah meh-dee-**see**-nah **pah**-rah lah **ahl**-tah preh-see-**ohn**?

Do you take medicine to thin your blood?

¿Toma medicina para hacer menos espesa la sangre?
Toh-mah meh-dee-**see**-nah **pah**-rah ah-**sehr meh**-nohs ehs-**peh**-sah lah **sahn**-greh?

Do you take aspirin?

¿Toma aspirina?
Toh-mah ahs-pee-**ree**-nah?

Do you take Coumadin?

¿Toma Coumadina?
Toh-mah koo-mah-**dee**-nah?

Do you have problems with your blood clotting?

¿Tiene problemas con la coagulación de la sangre?
Tee-**eh**-neh proh-**bleh**-mahs kohn lah koh-ah-goo-lah-see-**ohn** deh lah **sahn**-greh?

Do you have problems with your liver?

¿Tiene problemas con el hígado?
Tee-**eh**-neh proh-**bleh**-mahs kohn ehl **ee**-gah-doh?

Do you drink alcohol?

¿Toma alcohol?
Toh-mah ahl-**kohl**?

Do you feel dizzy?	¿Se siente mareado / -a? Seh see-**ehn**-teh mah-reh-**ah**-doh / -dah?
Do you have a headache?	¿Tiene dolor de cabeza? Tee-**eh**-neh doh-**lohr** deh kah-**beh**-sah?
Do you have chest pain?	¿Tiene dolor en el pecho? Tee-**eh**-neh doh-**lohr** ehn ehl **peh**-choh?

Common Phrases for the Exam for Epistaxis

Put your head forward and pinch your nose.	Ponga su cabeza hacia enfrente y apriete la nariz. **Pohn**-gah soo kah-**beh**-sah **ah**-see-ah ehn-**frehn**-teh ee ah-pree-**eh**-teh lah nah-**rees**.
Breathe through your mouth.	Respire por la boca. Rehs-**pee**-reh pohr lah **boh**-kah.
Do not put your head back.	No ponga la cabeza hacia atrás. Noh **pohn**-gah lah kah-**beh**-sah **ah**-see-ah ah-**tras**.
Block a side of your nose and blow.	Tape un lado de las nariz y sople. **Tah**-peh oon **lah**-doh deh lah nah-**rees** ee **soh**-pleh.
I need to pack your nose.	Necesito empacar su nariz. Neh-seh-**see**-toh ehm-pah-**kahr** soo nah-**rees**.

Discharge Instructions for Epistaxis

See your doctor tomorrow to remove the packing.

Vea a su médico mañana para que le quite el empaque.
Beh-ah ah soo **meh**-dee-koh mah-**nyah**-nah **pah**-rah keh leh **kee**-teh ehl ehm-**pah**-keh.

Do not blow your nose.

No se suene la nariz.
Noh seh **sweh**-neh lah nah-**rees.**

If the bleeding starts again, lean your head forward and pinch your nose for five minutes.

Si el sangrado comienza otra vez, incline su cabeza hacia enfrente y apriete la nariz por cinco minutos.
See ehl sahn-**grah**-doh koh-mee-**ehn**-sah **oh**-trah behs, een-**klee**-neh soo kah-**beh**-sah **ah**-see-ah ehn-**frehn**-teh ee ah-pree-**eh**-teh lah nah-**rees** pohr **seen**-koh mee-**noo**-tohs.

If the bleeding continues pinch your nose for five more minutes.

Si continúa el sangrado apriete la nariz por cinco minutos más.
See kohn-tee-**noo**-ah ehl sahn-**grah**-doh ah-pree-**eh**-teh lah nah-**rees** pohr **seen**-koh mee-**noo**-tohs mahs.

Go to the hospital if the bleeding continues for more than 15 minutes.

Vaya al hospital si el sangrado continúa por más de 15 minutos.
Bah-yah ahl ohs-pee-**tahl** see ehl sahn-**grah**-doh kohn-tee-**noo**-ah pohr mahs deh **keen**-seh mee-**noo**-tohs.

Neck Pain

Dolor del Cuello

Doh-**lohr** dehl **kweh**-yoh

Show me where you have the pain.

Enséñeme dónde tiene el dolor.
Ehn-**seh**-nyeh-meh **dohn**-deh tee-**eh**-neh ehl doh-**lohr**.

For how many days have you had the pain?

¿Por cuántos días ha tenido el dolor?
Pohr **kwahn**-tohs **dee**-ahs ah teh-**nee**-doh ehl doh-**lohr**?

Did you receive a blow to the neck?

¿Recibió un golpe al cuello?
Reh-see-bee-**oh** oon **gohl**-peh ahl **kweh**-yoh?

Did you receive a blow to the head?

¿Recibió un golpe a la cabeza?
Reh-see-bee-**oh** oon **gohl**-peh ah lah kah-**beh**-sah?

Did you fall?

¿Se cayó?
Seh kah-**yoh**?

Were you in an auto accident?

¿Estuvo en un accidente?
Ehs-**too**-boh ehn oon ak-see-**dehn**-teh?

Does the pain travel to your shoulders (arms)?

¿Le viaja el dolor hacia los hombros (brazos)?
Leh bee-**ah**-hah ehl doh-**lohr** **ah**-see-ah lohs **ohm**-bros (**brah**-sohs)?

Do you feel numbness in your arms?

¿Siente entumidos los brazos?
See-**ehn**-teh ehn-too-**mee**-dohs lohs **brah**-sohs?

Do you have pain when you move your head to the right (left)?

¿Tiene dolor al mover la cabeza hacia la derecha (izquierda)?

Tee-**eh**-neh doh-**lohr** ahl moh-**behr** lah kah-**beh**-sah **ah**-see-ah lah deh-**reh**-chah (ees-kee-**ehr**-dah)?

Do you have difficulty turning your head?

¿Tiene dificultad para voltear su cabeza?

Tee-**eh**-neh dee-fee-kool-**tahd pah**-rah bohl-teh-**ahr** soo kah-**beh**-sah?

Do you have a fever?

¿Tiene fiebre?

Tee-**eh**-neh fee-**eh**-breh?

Do you have dizzy spells?

¿Tiene mareos?

Tee-**eh**-neh mah-**reh**-ohs?

Do you have nausea or vomiting?

¿Tiene náusea o vómito?

Tee-**eh**-neh **nah**-oo-seh-ah oh **boh**-mee-toh?

Do you have a sore throat?

¿Tiene dolor de garganta?

Tee-**eh**-neh doh-**lohr** deh gahr-**gahn**-tah?

Does it feel like your neck is twisted to one side?

¿Siente como si tuviera el cuello torcido hacia un lado?

See-**ehn**-teh **koh**-moh see too-**bee**-eh-rah ehl **kweh**-yoh tohr-**see**-doh **ah**-see-ah oon **lah**-doh?

Do you have problems keeping your balance?

¿Tiene problemas para mantener su balance?

Tee-**eh**-neh proh-**bleh**-mahs **pah**-rah mahn-teh-**nehr** soo bah-**lahn**-seh?

Common Phrases for the Exam for Neck Pain

I need to examine your neck.

Necesito examinarle el cuello.
Neh-seh-**see**-toh ek-sah-mee-**nahr**-leh ehl **kweh**-yoh.

Try to touch your chest with your chin.

Trate de tocar su pecho con su mentón.
Trah-teh deh toh-**kahr** soo **peh**-choh kohn soo mehn-**tohn**.

Move your head back.

Mueva la cabeza hacia atrás.
Mweh-bah lah kah-**beh**-sah **ah**-see-ah ah-**trahs**.

Turn your head to the right (left).

Voltee la cabeza hacia la derecha (izquierda).
Bohl-**teh**-eh lah kah-**beh**-sah **ah**-see-ah lah deh-**reh**-chah (ees-kee-**ehr**-dah).

I need to take some X rays of your neck.

Es necesario sacarle unas radiografías del cuello.
Ehs neh-seh-**sah**-ree-oh sah-**kahr**-leh **oo**-nahs rah-dee-oh-grah-**fee**-ahs dehl **kweh**-yoh.

I need to get a CT of your neck.

Es necesario sacarle un CT del cuello.
Ehs neh-seh-**sah**-ree-oh sah-**kahr**-leh oon seh teh dehl **kweh**-yoh.

You have muscle spasm in your neck.

Usted tiene espasmo muscular en el cuello.
Oos-**tehd** tee-**eh**-neh ehs-**pahs**-moh moos-koo-**lahr** ehn ehl **kweh**-yoh.

You have a fracture.

Usted tiene una fractura.
Oos-**tehd** tee-**eh**-neh **oo**-nah frak-**too**-rah.

You have a strain.	Usted tiene una torcedura. Oos-**tehd** tee-**eh**-neh **oo**-nah tohr-seh-**doo**-rah.
You need a muscle relaxer.	Necesita un relajante muscular. Neh-seh-**see**-tah oon reh-lah-**han**-teh moos-koo-**lahr**.

Discharge Instructions for Neck Pain

Fill a plastic bag with ice and place it on your neck for half an hour every six hours for two days.

Llene con hielo una bolsa de plástico y póngala en su cuello por media hora cada seis horas por dos días. **Yeh**-neh kohn **yeh**-loh **oo**-nah **bohl**-sah deh **plahs**-tee-koh ee **pohn**-gah-lah ehn soo **kweh**-yoh pohr **meh**-dee-ah **oh**-rah **kah**-dah **seh**-ees **oh**-rahs pohr dohs **dee**-ahs.

You can also use a moist hot towel. Place it on your neck for half an hour every six hours.

También puede usar una toalla mojada con agua caliente. Póngala en su cuello por media hora cada seis horas. Tahm-bee-**ehn pweh**-deh oo-**sahr oo**-nah toh-**ah**-yah moh-**hah**-dah kohn **ah**-gwah kah-lee-**ehn**-teh. **Pohn**-gah-lah ehn soo **kweh**-yoh pohr **meh**-dee-ah **oh**-rah **kah**-dah **seh**-ees **oh**-rahs pohr dohs **dee**-ahs.

Take your medication.

Tome su medicina. **Toh**-meh soo meh-dee-**see**-nah.

Come back if you don't feel better or if you feel worse.

Regrese si no mejora o si está peor.

Reh-**greh**-seh see noh meh-**hoh**-rah oh see ehs-**tah** peh-**ohr**.

Part B
Cardiovascular/Respiratory

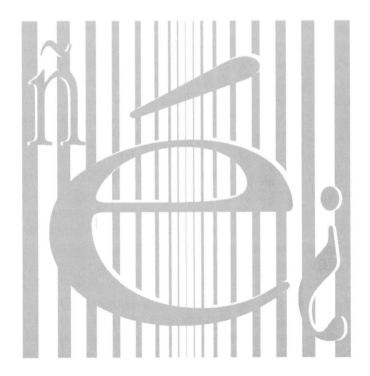

Chest Pain

Dolor del Pecho

Doh-**lohr** dehl **peh**-choh

Point to where the pain is, please.

Apunte dónde tiene el dolor, por favor.
Ah-**poon**-teh **dohn**-deh tee-**eh**-neh ehl doh-**lohr**, pohr fah-**bohr**.

Do you have pain in the middle of your chest?

¿Tiene dolor en medio del pecho?
Tee-**eh**-neh doh-**lohr** ehn **meh**-dee-oh dehl **peh**-choh?

Do you have pain in the right (left) side of your chest?

¿Tiene dolor en el lado derecho (izquierdo) del pecho?
Tee-**eh**-neh doh-**lohr** ehn ehl **lah**-doh deh-**reh**-choh (ees-kee-**ehr**-doh) dehl **peh**-choh?

Do you have pain in the pit of your stomach?

¿Tiene dolor en la boca del estómago?
Tee-**eh**-neh doh-**lohr** ehn lah **boh**-kah dehl ehs-**toh**-mah-goh?

Do you have pain over your entire chest?

¿Tiene dolor en todo el pecho?
Tee-**eh**-neh doh-**lohr** ehn **toh**-doh ehl **peh**-choh?

When did the pain start?

¿Cuándo empezó el dolor?
Kwahn-doh ehm-peh-**soh** ehl doh-**lohr**?

(X) minutes ago.

(X) minutos.
(X) mee-**noo**-tohs.

| (X) hours ago. | (X) horas. |
| | (X) **oh**-rahs. |

| (X) days ago. | (X) días. |
| | (X) **dee**-ahs. |

| Have you had this type of pain before? | ¿Ha tenido este tipo de dolor antes? |
| | Ah teh-**nee**-doh ehs-teh **tee**-poh deh doh-**lohr ahn**-tehs? |

| How long does the pain last? | ¿Cuánto tiempo le dura el dolor? |
| | **Kwahn**-toh tee-**ehm**-poh leh **doo**-rah ehl doh-**lohr**? |

| Is it constant? | ¿Es constante? |
| | Ehs kohn-**stahn**-teh? |

| (X) seconds. | (X) segundos. |
| | (X) seh-**goon**-dohs. |

| (X) minutes. | (X) minutos. |
| | (X) mee-**noo**-tohs. |

| (X) hours. | (X) horas. |
| | (X) **oh**-rahs. |

| How many times a day do you get the pain? | ¿Cuántas veces le da el dolor al día? |
| | **Kwahn**-tahs **beh**-sehs leh dah ehl doh-**lohr** ahl **dee**-ah? |

| Does the pain travel to your left shoulder (arm)? | ¿Le viaja el dolor al hombro (brazo) izquierdo? |
| | Leh bee-**ah**-hah ehl doh-**lohr** ahl **ohm**-broh (**brah**-soh) ees-kee-**ehr**-doh? |

| Does the pain travel to your neck? | ¿Le viaja el dolor al cuello? |
| | Leh bee-**ah**-hah ehl doh-**lohr** ahl **kweh**-yoh? |

Does the pain travel to your jaw (back)?

¿Le viaja el dolor a la mandíbula (espalda)?
Leh bee-**ah**-hah ehl doh-**lohr** ah lah mahn-**dee**-boo-lah (ehs-**pahl**-dah)?

What is the pain like?

¿Cómo es el dolor?
Koh-moh ehs ehl doh-**lohr**?

Is it acute / sharp?

¿Es agudo?
Ehs ah-**goo**-doh?

Is it severe?

¿Es severo?
Ehs seh-**beh**-roh?

Is it piercing?

¿Es punzante?
Ehs poon-**sahn**-teh?

Is it like a knife?

¿Es como cuchillo?
Ehs **koh**-moh koo-**chee**-yoh?

Does it ache?

¿Es adolorido?
Ehs ah-doh-loh-**ree**-doh?

Is it like a pressure?

¿Es opresivo?
Ehs oh-preh-**see**-boh?

Does it burn?

¿Es quemante?
Ehs keh-**mahn**-teh?

Does it throb?

¿Es pulsante / latiendo?
Ehs pool-**sahn**-teh / lah-tee-ehn-doh?

Does the pain occur when you are sitting or lying down?

¿Le da el dolor cuando está sentado / -a o acostado / -a?
Leh dah ehl doh-**lohr kwahn**-doh ehs-**tah** sehn-**tah**-doh / -dah oh ah-kohs-**tah**-doh / -dah?

Is the pain better if you lean forward?	¿Le mejora el dolor si se inclina hacia adelante? Leh meh-**ho**-rah ehl doh-**lohr** see seh een-**klee**-nah **ah**-see-ah ah-deh-**lahn**-teh?
Is the pain worse if you lie down?	¿Le empeora el dolor si se acuesta? Leh ehm-peh-**oh**-rah ehl doh-**lohr** see seh ah-**kwehs**-tah?
Do you have the pain when you walk?	¿Le da el dolor cuando camina? Leh dah ehl doh-**lohr kwahn**-doh kah-**mee**-nah?
After walking how many blocks do you get the pain?	¿Después de caminar cuántas cuadras le da el dolor? Dehs-**pwehs** deh kah-mee-**nahr kwahn**-tahs **kwah**-drahs leh dah ehl doh-**lohr**?
If you get the pain when you walk, do you keep walking?	Si le da el dolor cuando camina, ¿sigue caminando? See leh dah ehl doh-**lohr kwahn**-doh kah-**mee**-nah, **see**-geh kah-mee-**nahn**-doh?
Does the pain go away after you rest (stop walking)?	¿Se le quita el dolor después de descansar (dejar de caminar)? Seh leh **kee**-tah ehl doh-**lohr** dehs-**pwehs** deh dehs-kahn-**sahr** (deh-**har** deh kah-mee-**nahr**)?
When you have pain do you feel short of breath?	¿Cuando tiene dolor siente falta de aire? **Kwahn**-doh tee-**eh**-neh doh-**lohr** see-**ehn**-teh **fahl**-tah deh **ah**-ee-reh?

When you have pain do you get nausea or vomiting?

¿Cuando tiene dolor le da náusea o vómito?
Kwahn-doh tee-**eh**-neh doh-**lohr** leh dah **nah**-oo-seh-ah oh **boh**-mee-toh?

Do you sweat with the pain?

¿Suda con el dolor?
Soo-dah kohn ehl doh-**lohr**?

Do you feel a choking sensation in your neck?

¿Se siente sofocado / a en el cuello?
Seh see-**ehn**-teh soh-foh-**kah**-doh / -dah ehn ehl **kweh**-yoh?

What gives you chest pain?

¿Qué actividades o cosas le producen el dolor?
Keh ahk-tee-bee-**dah**-dehs oh **koh**-sahs leh proh-**doo**-sehn ehl doh-**lohr**?

Walking in the street?

¿Caminar en la calle?
Kah-mee-**nahr** ehn lah **kah**-yeh?

Walking up stairs?

¿Subir escaleras?
Soo-**beer** ehs-kah-**leh**-rahs?

Coughing?

¿Toser?
Toh-**sehr**?

Taking a deep breath?

¿Respirar profundo?
Rehs-pee-**rahr** proh-**foon**-doh?

Eating spicy or fried food?

¿La comida picante o frita?
Lah koh-**mee**-dah pee-**kahn**-teh oh **free**-tah?

Emotional upset?

¿El enojo emocional?
Ehl eh-**noh**-ho eh-moh-see-oh-**nahl**?

Have you taken something for the pain?	¿Ha tomado algo para el dolor? Ah toh-**mah**-doh **ahl**-goh **pah**-rah ehl doh-**lohr**?
Have you taken . . .	¿Ha tomado... Ah toh-**mah**-doh...
sublingual nitroglycerin?	nitroglicerina debajo de la lengua? nee-troh-glee-seh-**ree**-nah deh-**bah**-hoh deh lah **lehn**-gwah?
antacids?	antiácidos? ahn-tee-**ah**-see-dohs?
How many nitroglycerin pills did you take today?	¿Cuántas pastillas de nitroglicerina ha tomado hoy? **Kwahn**-tahs pahs-**tee**-yahs deh nee-troh-glee-seh-**ree**-nah ah toh-**mah**-doh **oh**-ee?
Did your pain go away after taking nitroglycerin?	¿Se le quitó el dolor después de tomar la nitroglicerina? Seh leh kee-**toh** ehl doh-**lohr** dehs-**pwehs** deh toh-**mahr** lah nee-troh-glee-seh-**ree**-nah?
Do you have angina?	¿Tiene angina de pecho? Tee-**eh**-neh ahn-**hee**-nah deh **peh**-choh?
Do you have a fever?	¿Tiene fiebre? Tee-**eh**-neh fee-**eh**-breh?
Do you have a cough?	¿Tiene tos? Tee-**eh**-neh tohs?

If you have a cough, do you have phlegm?	¿Si tiene tos, le sale flema? See tee-**eh**-neh tohs, leh **sah**-leh **fleh**-mah?
What color is the phlegm?	¿De qué color es la flema? Deh **keh** koh-**lohr** ehs lah **fleh**-mah?
Is it clear?	¿Es clara? Ehs **klah**-rah?
Is it yellow?	¿Es amarilla? Ehs ah-mah-**ree**-yah?
Is it green?	¿Es verde? Ehs **behr**-deh?
Is it red?	¿Es roja? Ehs **roh**-hah?
How many pillows do you use to sleep?	¿Cuántas almohadas usa usted para dormir? **Kwahn**-tahs ahl-moh-**ah**-dahs **oo**-sah oos-**tehd pah**-rah dohr-**meer**?
Did your feet or ankles swell up?	¿Se le hinchan los pies o los tobillos? Seh leh-**een**-chan lohs pee-**ehs** oh lohs toh-**bee**-yohs?
Do you wake up at night because of shortness of breath?	¿Se levanta durante la noche por falta de aire? Seh leh-**bahn**-tah doo-**rahn**-teh lah **noh**-cheh pohr **fahl**-tah deh **ah**-ee-reh?
Do you have high blood pressure?	¿Tiene usted alta presión de la sangre? Tee-**eh**-neh oos-**tehd ahl**-tah preh-see-**ohn** deh lah **sahn**-greh?

Do you take high blood pressure medication?	¿Toma medicina para la alta presión? **Toh**-mah meh-dee-**see**-nah **pah**-rah lah **ahl**-tah preh-see-**ohn**?
Do you have diabetes?	¿Tiene usted diabetes? Tee-**eh**-neh oos-**tehd** dee-ah-**beh**-tehs?
Did any member of your family (such as your father, brother, or uncle) die of heart trouble before age 50?	¿Algún miembro de su familia (como su padre, hermano o tío) se murio del corazón antes de los 50 años? Ahl-**goon** mee-**ehm**-broh deh soo fah-**mee**-lee-ah (**koh**-moh soo **pah**-dreh, ehr-**mah**-noh oh **tee**-oh) seh moo-ree-**oh** dehl koh-rah-**sohn ahn**-tehs deh los seen-**kwehn**-tah **ah**-nyohs?
Do you smoke?	¿Fuma usted? **Foo**-mah oos-**tehd**?
For how many years?	¿Por cuántos años? Pohr **kwahn**-tohs **ah**-nyohs?
How many cigarettes do you smoke a day?	¿Cuántos cigarrillos fuma por día? **Kwahn**-tohs see-gah-**ree**-yohs **foo**-mah pohr **dee**-ah?
Have you had an angiogram?	¿Ha tenido un angiograma? Ah teh-**nee**-doh oon ahn-gee-oh-**grah**-mah?

Have they told you if you have a blockage in your coronary arteries?	¿Le han dicho si usted tiene bloqueos en las arterias del corazón? Leh ahn **dee**-choh see oos-**tehd** tee-**eh**-neh bloh-**keh**-ohs ehn lahs ahr-**teh**-ree-ahs dehl koh-rah-**sohn**?
Have you ever had a heart attack or infarct in the past?	¿Ha tenido ataque del corazón o infarto en el pasado? Ah teh-**nee**-doh ah-**tah**-keh dehl koh-rah-**sohn** oh een-**fahr**-toh ehn ehl pah-**sah**-doh?
Do you know if you have high cholesterol?	Sabe si tiene el colesterol alto? Sah-beh see tee-**eh**-neh ehl koh-lehs-teh-**rohl ahl**-toh?
Have you had a stress test?	¿Ha tenido una prueba del esfuerzo? Ah teh-**nee**-doh **oo**-nah **prweh**-bah dehl ehs-**fwehr**-soh?
How many minutes did you last on the exam?	¿Cuántos minutos pudo durar con el examen? **Kwahn**-tohs mee-**noo**-tohs **poo**-doh doo-**rahr** kohn ehl ek-**sah**-mehn?

Common Phrases for the Exam for Chest Pain

Show me where the pain is.	Muéstreme dónde tiene el dolor. **Mwehs**-treh-meh **dohn**-deh tee-**eh**-neh ehl doh-**lohr**.
I am going to examine your heart.	Le voy a examinar el corazón. Leh boy ah ek-sah-mee-**nahr** ehl koh-rah-**sohn**.

I am going to examine your lungs.	Le voy a examinar los pulmones. Leh boy ah ek-sah-mee-**nahr** lohs pool-**mohn**-ehs.
Take a deep breath.	Respire profundo. Rehs-**pee**-reh proh-**foon**-doh.
Take a deep breath and hold it.	Tome una respiración profunda y mantenga el aire. **Toh**-meh **oo**-nah rehs-pee-rah-see-**ohn** proh-**foon**-dah ee mahn-**tehn**-gah ehl **ah**-ee-reh.
You have angina.	Usted tiene angina del pecho. Oos-**tehd** tee-**eh**-neh ahn-**hee**-nah dehl **peh**-choh.
You had a heart attack (an infarct).	Usted tuvo un ataque cardíaco (un infarto en el corazón). Oos-**tehd too**-boh oon ah-**tah**-keh kahr-**dee**-ah-koh (oon een-**fahr**-toh ehn ehl koh-rah-**sohn**).
You have heart failure (water in the lungs).	Usted tiene falla del corazón (agua en los pulmones). Oos-**tehd** tee-**eh**-neh **fah**-yah dehl koh-rah-**sohn** (**ah**-gwah ehn lohs pool-**mohn**-ehs).
You have pneumonia.	Usted tiene pulmonía. Oos-**tehd** tee-**eh**-neh pool-moh-**nee**-ah.
We need to do an electrocardiogram.	Necesitamos hacerle un electrocardiograma. Neh-seh-see-**tah**-mohs ah-**sehr**-leh oon eh-lek-troh-kahr-dee-oh-**grah**-mah.

We need to do blood tests.

Necesitamos hacerle análisis de sangre.
Neh-seh-see-**tah**-mohs ah-**sehr**-leh ah-**nah**-lee-sees deh **sahn**-greh.

We need to admit you to the hospital (in intensive care).

Vamos a internarlo en el hospital (en cuidado intensivo).
Bah-mohs ah een-tehr-**nahr**-loh ehn ehl ohs-pee-**tahl** (ehn kwi-**dah**-doh een-tehn-**see**-boh).

I am going to give you medicine under your tongue.

Voy a darle una medicina debajo de la lengua.
Boy ah **dahr**-leh **oo**-nah meh-dee-**see**-nah deh-**bah**-ho deh lah **lehn**-gwah.

Tell me if the pain goes away.

Dígame si le quita el dolor.
Dee-gah-meh see leh **kee**-tah ehl doh-**lohr**.

I am going to give you medicine to dissolve the blockage in the arteries of your heart.

Voy a darle medicina para disolver los bloqueos de las arterias de su corazón.
Boy ah **dahr**-leh meh-dee-**see**-nah **pah**-rah dee-sohl-**behr** lohs bloh-**keh**-ohs deh lahs ahr-**teh**-ree-ahs deh soo koh-rah-**sohn**.

Discharge Instructions for Chest Pain

Return to the hospital (clinic) if you have . . .

Regrese al hospital (a la clínica) si tiene...
Reh-**greh**-seh ahl ohs-pee-**tahl** (ah lah **klee**-nee-kah) see tee-**eh**-neh...

chest pain with shortness
of breath,

dolor en el pecho con
falta de aire,
doh-**lohr** ehn ehl **peh**-choh
kohn **fahl**-tah deh **ah**-ee-
reh,

chest pain with nausea,
vomiting or sweating,

dolor de pecho con
náusea, vómito o sudor,
doh-**lohr** deh **peh**-choh
kohn **nah**-oo-seh-ah, **boh**-
mee-toh oh soo-**dohr**,

pressure in your chest,

presión en el pecho,
preh-see-**ohn** ehn ehl **peh**-
choh,

or if you have dizziness
with the chest pain.

o mareos con el dolor de
pecho.
oh mah-**reh**-ohs kohn ehl
doh-**lohr** deh **peh**-choh.

If you have chest pain, put a
pill under your tongue every
five minutes.

Si tiene dolor tome una
pastilla debajo de su lengua
cada cinco minutos.
See tee-**eh**-neh doh-**lohr** toh-
meh **oo**-nah pahs-**tee**-yah deh-
bah-ho deh soo **lehn**-gwah
kah-dah **seen**-koh mee-**noo**-
tohs.

If the pain does not go
away after three pills
return to the hospital
(clinic).

Si no se le quita el dolor
después de tomar tres
pastillas regrese al
hospital (a la clínica).
See noh seh leh **kee**-tah
ehl doh-**lohr** dehs-**pwehs**
deh toh-**mahr** trehs pahs-
tee-yahs reh-**greh**-seh ahl
ohs-pee-**tahl** (ah lah **klee**-
nee-kah).

Cough and Shortness of Breath

Tos y Falta de Aire

Tohs ee **fahl**-tah deh **ah**-ee-reh

Do you have a cough?	¿Tiene tos? Tee-**eh**-neh tohs?
How many days have you had a cough?	¿Por cuántos días ha tenido la tos? Pohr **kwahn**-tohs **dee**-ahs ah teh-**nee**-doh lah tohs?
Do you have phlegm when you cough?	¿Le sale flema cuando tose? Leh **sah**-leh **fleh**-mah **kwahn**-doh **toh**-seh?
What color is the phlegm?	¿De qué color es la flema? Deh keh koh-**lohr** ehs lah **fleh**-mah?
Is it clear?	¿Es clara? Ehs **klah**-rah?
Is it yellow?	¿Es amarilla? Ehs ah-mah-**ree**-yah?
Is it green?	¿Es verde? Ehs **behr**-deh?
Is it red?	¿Es roja? Ehs **roh**-hah?
Do you have fever?	¿Tiene fiebre o calentura? Tee-**eh**-neh fee-**eh**-breh oh kah-lehn-**too**-rah?
Do you have pain in your chest when you cough?	¿Le da dolor en el pecho cuando tose? Leh dah doh-**lohr** ehn ehl **peh**-choh **kwahn**-doh **toh**-seh?

Have you lost weight?

¿Ha perdido peso?
Ah pehr-**dee**-doh **peh**-soh?

How many pounds have you lost?

¿Cuántas libras ha perdido?
Kwahn-tahs **lee**-brahs ah pehr-**dee**-doh?

Do you sweat during the night?

¿Suda usted durante la noche?
Soo-dah oos-**tehd** doo-**rahn**-teh lah **noh**-cheh?

Do you have chills?

¿Tiene escalofríos?
Tee-**eh**-neh ehs-kah-loh-**free**-ohs?

Do you know if you have been in contact with a person with TB?

¿Sabe usted si ha tenido contacto con una persona con tuberculosis?
Sah-beh oos-**tehd** see ah teh-**nee**-doh kohn-**tak**-toh kohn **oo**-nah pehr-**soh**-nah kohn too-behr-koo-**loh**-sees?

Do you have shortness of breath?

¿Tiene falta de aire?
Tee-**eh**-neh **fahl**-tah deh **ah**-ee-reh?

Do you get short of breath when walking?

¿Le hace falta la respiración al caminar?
Leh **ah**-seh **fahl**-tah lah rehs-pee-rah-see-**ohn** ahl kah-mee-**nahr**?

After how many blocks?

¿Después de cuántas cuadras?
Dehs-**pwehs** deh **kwahn**-tahs **kwah**-drahs?

Do you have shortness of breath when you are sitting?	¿Tiene falta de aire cuando esta sentado / a? Tee-**eh**-neh **fahl**-tah deh **ah**-ee-reh **kwahn**-doh ehs-**tah** sehn-**tah**-doh / -dah?
Do you feel short of breath when you lie down?	¿Le hace falta la respiración cuando se acuesta? Le **ah**-seh **fahl**-tah lah rehs-pee-rah-see-**ohn** **kwahn**-doh seh ah-**kwehs**-tah?
Do you wake up at night with shortness of breath?	¿Se levanta usted durante la noche con falta de aire? Seh leh-**bahn**-tah oos-**tehd** doo-**rahn**-teh lah **noh**-cheh kohn **fahl**-tah deh **ah**-ee-reh?
How many pillows do you use to sleep?	¿Cuántas almohadas usa para dormir? **Kwahn**-tahs ahl-moh-**ah**-dahs **oo**-sah **pah**-rah dohr-**meer**?
Do your feet swell?	¿Se le hinchan los pies? Seh leh **een**-chan lohs pee-**ehs**?
Do you suffer from heart trouble?	¿Padece usted de problemas del corazón? Pah-**deh**-seh oos-**tehd** deh proh-**bleh**-mahs dehl koh-rah-**sohn**?
Do you suffer from asthma?	¿Padece usted de asma? Pah-**deh**-seh oos-**tehd** deh **ahs**-mah?

For how many years or months?	¿Por cuántos años o meses? Pohr **kwahn**-tohs **ah**-nyohs oh **meh**-sehs?
Do you smoke?	¿Fuma usted? **Foo**-mah oos-**tehd**?
How many cigarettes do you smoke a day?	¿Cuántos cigarrillos fuma por día? **Kwahn**-tohs see-gah-**ree**-yohs **foo**-mah pohr **dee**-ah?
For how many years?	¿Por cuántos años? Pohr **kwahn**-tohs **ah**-nyohs?
Do you take any medicine?	¿Toma usted algún medicamento? **Toh**-mah oos-**tehd** ahl-**goon** meh-dee-kah-**mehn**-toh?

Common Phrases for the Exam for Cough and Shortness of Breath

Breathe deeply, please.	Respire profundo, por favor. Rehs-**pee**-reh proh-**foon**-doh, pohr fah-**bohr**.
Put on your oxygen mask.	Póngase la máscara de oxígeno. **Pohn**-gah-seh lah **mahs**-kah-rah deh ohk-**see**-heh-noh.
We are going to take an X ray of your chest.	Vamos a sacarle una radiografía del pecho. **Bah**-mohs ah sah-**kahr**-leh oo-nah rah-dee-oh-grah-**fee**-ah dehl **peh**-choh.

You need a blood test.

Usted necesita análisis de sangre.
Oos-**tehd** neh-seh-**see**-tah ah-**nah**-lee-sehs deh **sahn**-greh.

We are going to draw blood from an artery to see if you need oxygen.

Vamos a sacarle sangre de una arteria para ver si usted necesita oxígeno.
Bah-mohs ah sah-**kahr**-leh **sahn**-greh deh **oo**-nah ahr-**teh**-ree-ah **pah**-rah behr see oos-**tehd** neh-seh-**see**-tah ohk-**see**-heh-noh.

We need a sample of your phlegm.

Necesitamos una muestra de flema.
Neh-seh-see-**tah**-mohs **oo**-nah **mwehs**-trah deh **fleh**-mah.

You need a treatment.

Usted necesita un tratamiento.
Oos-**tehd** neh-seh-**see**-tah oon trah-tah-mee-**ehn**-toh.

You have pneumonia.

Usted tiene pulmonía.
Oos-**tehd** tee-**eh**-neh pool-moh-**nee**-ah.

You have the flu (a cold).

Usted tiene gripe (catarro).
Oos-**tehd** tee-**eh**-neh **gree**-peh (kah-**tah**-roh).

You have asthma.

Usted tiene asma.
Oos-**tehd** tee-**eh**-neh **ahs**-mah.

You have tuberculosis.

Usted tiene tuberculosis.
Oos-**tehd** tee-**eh**-neh too-behr-koo-**loh**-sees.

Discharge Instructions for Cough and Shortness of Breath

Return to the hospital (clinic) if . . .

Regrese al hospital (a la clínica) si...
Reh-**greh**-seh ahl ohs-pee-**tahl** (ah lah **klee**-nee-kah) see...

you are still short of breath.

sigue con falta de aire.
see-geh kohn **fahl**-tah deh **ah**-ee-reh.

you are not getting better.

no se mejora.
noh seh meh-**hoh**-rah.

you have fever or vomiting.

tiene fiebre o vómito.
tee-**eh**-neh fee-**eh**-breh oh **boh**-mee-toh.

Stop smoking.

Deje de fumar.
Deh-he deh foo-**mahr**.

Take the medicine as indicated by your doctor.

Tome sus medicinas como le indicó el médico.
Toh-meh soos meh-dee-**see**-nahs **koh**-moh leh een-dee-**koh** ehl **meh**-dee-koh.

Hypertension

Alta Presion

Ahl-tah preh-see-**ohn**

Do you know if you have high blood pressure?

¿Sabe usted si tiene alta presión de la sangre?
Sah-beh oos-**tehd** see tee-**eh**-neh **ahl**-tah preh-see-**ohn** deh lah **sahn**-greh?

What medicine do you take?	¿Qué medicina toma? Keh meh-dee-**see**-nah **toh**-mah?
Do you take your medicine every day?	¿Toma usted su medicina todos los días? **Toh**-mah oos-**tehd** soo meh-dee-**see**-nah **toh**-dohs lohs **dee**-ahs?
When was the last time you took your medicine?	¿Cuándo fue la última vez que tomó su medicina? **Kwahn**-doh fweh lah **ool**-tee-mah vehs keh toh-**moh** soo meh-dee-**see**-nah?
(X) hours (days, weeks, months) ago.	(X) horas (días, semanas, meses). (X) **oh**-rahs (**dee**-ahs, seh-**mah**-nahs, **meh**-sehs).
Do you have a headache?	¿Tiene dolor de cabeza? Tee-**eh**-neh doh-**lohr** deh kah-**beh**-sah?
Where do you feel the pain?	¿Dónde siente el dolor? **Dohn**-deh see-**ehn**-teh ehl doh-**lohr**?
Does your forehead hurt?	¿Le duele la frente? Leh **dweh**-leh lah **frehn**-teh?
Does your temple hurt?	¿Le duele la sien? Leh **dweh**-leh lah see-**ehn**?
Does your occiput hurt?	¿Le duele el cerebro? Leh **dweh**-leh ehl seh-**reh**-broh?

Does your whole head hurt?	¿Le duele toda la cabeza?
	Leh **dweh**-leh **toh**-dah lah kah-**beh**-sah?
Do you have nausea or vomiting?	¿Tiene náusea o vómito?
	Tee-**eh**-neh **nah**-oo-seh-ah oh **boh**-mee-toh?
Do you have abdominal pain?	¿Tiene dolor en el abdomen?
	Tee-**eh**-neh doh-**lohr** ehn ehl ab-**doh**-mehn?
Do you have weakness in your hand (arm, leg, face)?	¿Tiene debilidad en la mano (el brazo, la pierna, la cara)?
	Tee-**eh**-neh deh-bee-lee-**dad** ehn lah **mah**-noh (ehl **brah**-soh, lah pee-**ehr**-nah, lah **kah**-rah)?
Do you have dizzy spells?	¿Tiene mareos?
	Tee-**eh**-neh mah-**reh**-ohs?
Do you have difficulty talking?	¿Tiene dificultad para hablar?
	Tee-**eh**-neh dee-fee-kool-**tahd** **pah**-rah ah-**blahr**?
Do you have chest pain?	¿Tiene dolor del pecho?
	Tee-**eh**-neh doh-**lohr** dehl **peh**-choh?
Do you have shortness of breath?	¿Tiene falta de aire?
	Tee-**eh**-neh **fahl**-tah deh **ah**-ee-reh?

Common Phrases for the Exam for Hypertension

Your blood pressure is very high.	Usted tiene la presión de sangre muy alta.
	Oos-**tehd** tee-**eh**-neh lah preh-see-**ohn** deh **sahn**-greh **moo**-ee **ahl**-tah.

We are going to give you medicine to lower your blood pressure.	Le vamos a dar medicina para bajarle la presión. Leh **bah**-mohs ah dahr meh-dee-**see**-nah **pah**-rah bah-**har**-leh lah preh-see-**ohn**.
You need an EKG.	Usted necesita un electrocardiograma. Oos-**tehd** neh-seh-**see**-tah oon eh-lek-troh-kar-dee-oh-**grah**-mah.
You need a CT scan.	Usted necesita un CT. Oos-**tehd** neh-seh-**see**-tah oon seh teh.
You need blood and urine tests.	Usted necesita pruebas de sangre y orina. Oos-**tehd** neh-seh-**see**-tah **prweh**-bahs deh **sahn**-greh ee oh-**ree**-nah.
We are going to admit you.	Lo / La vamos a internar. Loh / Lah **bah**-mohs ah een-tehr-**nahr**.

Discharge Instructions for Hypertension

Take your medicine as indicated.	Tome su medicina como le indicaron. **Toh**-meh soo meh-dee-**see**-nah **koh**-moh leh een-dee-**kah**-rohn.
Return to the hospital (clinic) if you have . . .	Regrese al hospital (a la clínica) si tiene... Reh-**greh**-seh ahl ohs-pee-**tahl** (ah lah **klee**-nee-kah) see tee-**eh**-neh...

severe headaches,	dolores de cabeza severos, doh-**loh**-rehs deh kah-**beh**-sah seh-**beh**-rohs,
dizziness,	mareos, mah-**reh**-ohs,
weakness in your hand, arm or leg,	debilidad en la mano, el brazo o la pierna, deh-bee-lee-**dad** ehn lah **mah**-noh, ehl **brah**-soh oh lah pee-**ehr**-nah,
or chest pain.	o dolor del pecho. oh doh-**lohr** dehl **peh**-choh.

Congestive Heart Failure

Insuficiencia Cardíaca
Een-soo-fee-see-**ehn**-see-ah kahr-**dee**-ah-kah

Since when have you been short of breath?	¿Desde cuándo tiene falta de aire? **Dehs**-deh kwahn-doh tee-**eh**-neh **fahl**-tah deh ah-ee-reh?
For (X) hours (days, weeks).	Desde (X) horas (días, semanas). **Dehs**-deh (X) **oh**-rahs (**dee**-ahs, seh-**mah**-nahs).
Did the shortness of breath start little by little?	¿Empezó la falta de aire poco a poco? Ehm-peh-**soh** lah **fahl**-tah deh ah-ee-reh **poh**-koh a **poh**-koh?

Did the shortness of breath start suddenly?	¿Empezó la falta de aire de repente? Ehm-peh-**soh** lah **fahl**-tah deh **ah**-ee-reh deh reh-**pehn**-teh?
How many blocks can you walk without feeling short of breath?	¿Cuántas cuadras puede caminar sin tener falta de aire? **Kwahn**-tahs **kwah**-drahs **pweh**-deh kah-mee-**nahr** seen teh-**nehr fahl**-tah deh **ah**-ee-reh?
Were you able to walk farther last week?	¿Podía caminar mas lejos la semana pasada? Poh-**dee**-ah kah-mee-**nahr** mahs **leh**-hos lah seh-**mah**-nah pah-**sah**-dah?
How many blocks were you able to walk?	¿Cuántas cuadras podía caminar? **Kwahn**-tahs **kwah**-drahs poh-**dee**-ah kah-mee-**nahr**?
Do your ankles or feet swell?	¿Se le hinchan los tobillos o los pies? Seh leh **een**-chan lohs toh-**bee**-yohs oh lohs pee-**ehs**?
Do you wake up at night short of breath?	¿Se levanta usted en la noche por falta de aire? Seh leh-**bahn**-tah oos-**tehd** ehn lah **noh**-cheh pohr **fahl**-tah deh **ah**-ee-reh?
How many pillows do you use to sleep?	¿Cuántas almohadas usa usted para dormir? **Kwahn**-tahs ahl-moh-**ah**-dahs **oo**-sah oos-**tehd pah**-rah dohr-**meer**?

How many pillows did you use before?	¿Cuántas almohadas usaba usted antes? **Kwahn**-tahs ahl-moh-**ah**-dahs oo-**sah**-bah oos-**tehd ahn**-tehs?
Do you feel short of breath when you walk or go up stairs?	¿Siente falta de aire al caminar o subir escaleras? See-**ehn**-teh **fahl**-tah deh **ah**-ee-reh ahl kah-mee-**nahr** oh soo-**beer** ehs-kah-**leh**-rahs?
Have you had congestive heart failure (fluid in the lungs) before?	¿Ha tenido insuficiencia cardíaca (líquido en los pulmones) antes? Ah teh-**nee**-doh een-soo-fee-see-**ehn**-see-ah kahr-**dee**-ah-kah (**lee**-kee-doh ehn lohs pool-**moh**-nehs) **ahn**-tehs?
Do you take a diuretic (water pill)?	¿Toma usted diurético (pastilla de agua)? **Toh**-mah oos-**tehd** dee-oo-**reh**-tee-koh (pahs-**tee**-yah deh ah-**gwah**)?
When was the last time you took your medicine?	¿Cuándo fue la última vez que tomó su medicina? **Kwahn**-doh fweh lah **ool**-tee-mah behs keh toh-**moh** soo meh-dee-**see**-nah?
Did you take it today?	¿La tomó hoy? Lah toh-**moh oh**-ee?
Did you take it yesterday?	¿La tomó ayer? Lah toh-**moh** ah-**yehr**?
Have you had chest pain?	¿Ha tenido dolor del pecho? Ah teh-**nee**-doh doh-**lohr** dehl **peh**-choh?

Have you had pressure in the chest?	¿Ha tenido presión en el pecho? Ah teh-**nee**-doh preh-see-**ohn** ehn ehl **peh**-choh?
Do you have chest pain now?	¿Tiene dolor de pecho ahora? Tee-**eh**-neh doh-**lohr** deh **peh**-choh ah-**oh**-rah?

Common Phrases for the Exam for Congestive Heart Failure

You need a chest X ray.	Usted necesita una radiografía del pecho. Oos-**tehd** neh-seh-**see**-tah **oo**-nah rah-dee-oh-grah-**fee**-ah dehl **peh**-choh.
You need an EKG.	Usted necesita un electrocardiograma. Oos-**tehd** neh-seh-**see**-tah oon eh-lek-troh-kar-dee-oh-**grah**-mah.
I need to put a catheter in your bladder.	Necesito ponerle una sonda en la vejiga. Neh-seh-**see**-toh poh-**nehr**-leh **oo**-nah **sohn**-dah ehn lah beh-**hee**-gah.
I am going to give you a diuretic by vein.	Le voy a dar un diurético por la vena. Leh **boh**-ee ah dahr oon dee-oo-**reh**-tee-koh pohr lah **beh**-nah.
You have a lot of fluid in the lungs.	Usted tiene mucho líquido en los pulmones. Oos-**tehd** tee-**eh**-neh **moo**-choh **lee**-kee-doh ehn lohs pool-**mohn**-ehs.

You have had a heart attack.	Usted ha tenido un ataque del corazón.
	Oos-**tehd** ah teh-**nee**-doh oon ah-**tah**-keh dehl koh-rah-**sohn**.
We need to admit you.	Necesitamos internarlo / la.
	Neh-seh-see-**tah**-mohs een-tehr-**nahr**-loh / -lah.

Discharge Instructions for Congestive Heart Failure

Take one pill of your medicine every (X) hours.	Tome una pastilla de su medicina cada (X) horas.
	Toh-meh **oo**-nah pahs-**tee**-yah deh soo meh-dee-**see**-nah **kah**-dah (X) **oh**-rahs.
Avoid salt.	Evite la sal.
	Eh-**bee**-teh lah sahl.
Return to the hospital (clinic) if . . .	Regrese al hospital (a la clínica) si...
	Reh-**greh**-seh ahl ohs-pee-**tahl** (ah lah **klee**-nee-kah) see...
you have shortness of breath,	tiene falta de aire,
	tee-**eh**-neh **fahl**-tah deh **ah**-ee-reh,
you have chest pain,	tiene dolor del pecho,
	tee-**eh**-neh doh-**lohr** dehl **peh**-choh,
your ankles or feet swell.	se le hinchan los tobillos o pies.
	seh leh **een**-chan lohs toh-**bee**-yohs o pee-**ehs**.

Asthma

Asma

Ahs-mah

Is this asthma attack worse than the others?

¿Es este ataque de asma peor que los otros?
Ehs **ehs**-teh ah-**tah**-keh deh **ahs**-mah peh-**ohr** keh lohs **oh**-trohs?

When did you start getting short of breath?

¿Cuándo empezó la falta de aire?
Kwahn-doh ehm-peh-**soh** lah **fahl**-tah deh **ah**-ee-reh?

Do you have a cough?

¿Tiene tos?
Tee-**eh**-neh tohs?

Does phlegm come out when you cough?

¿Le sale flema cuando tose?
Leh **sah**-leh **fleh**-mah **kwahn**-doh **toh**-seh?

What color is the phlegm?

¿De qué color es la flema?
Deh **keh** koh-**lohr** ehs lah **fleh**-mah?

Is it clear?

¿Es clara?
Ehs **klah**-rah?

Is it yellow?

¿Es amarilla?
Ehs ah-mah-**ree**-yah?

Is it green?

¿Es verde?
Ehs **behr**-deh?

Do you have chest pain?

¿Tiene dolor del pecho?
Tee-**eh**-neh doh-**lohr** dehl **peh**-choh?

Does your chest hurt when you cough or take a deep breath?

¿Le duele el pecho cuando tose o respira profundo?
Leh **dweh**-leh ehl **peh**-choh **kwahn**-doh **toh**-seh oh rehs-**pee**-rah proh-**foon**-doh?

Do you have fever?

¿Tiene fiebre?
Tee-**eh**-neh fee-**eh**-breh?

Do you have nausea or vomiting?

¿Tiene náusea o vómito?
Tee-**eh**-neh **nah**-oo-seh-ah oh **boh**-mee-toh?

Have you taken medicine today for the asthma?

¿Ha tomado alguna medicina para el asma hoy?
Ah toh-**mah**-doh ahl-**goo**-nah meh-dee-**see**-nah **pah**-rah ehl **ahs**-mah **oh**-ee?

What medicine do you take?

¿Qué medicina toma?
Keh meh-dee-**see**-nah **toh**-mah?

Theophylline?

¿Teofilina?
Teh-oh-fee-**lee**-nah?

Prednisone?

¿Prednisona?
Prehd-nee-**soh**-nah?

Azmacort?

¿Azmacort?
Asma-**kohrt**?

Proventil?

¿Proventil?
Proh-behn-**teel**?

Ventolin?

¿Ventolin?
Behn-toh-**leen**?

Alupent?

¿Alupent?
Ah-loo-**pehnt**?

Do you use an inhaler?

¿Usa un inhalador?
Oo-sah oon een-ah-lah-**dor**?

How many times have you used your inhaler today?

¿Cuántas veces ha usado su inhalador hoy?
Kwahn-tahs **beh**-sehs ah oo-**sah**-doh soo een-ah-lah-**dohr oh**-ee?

Have you taken Prednisone in the past?

¿Ha tomado Prednisona en el pasado?
Ah toh-**mah**-doh prehd-nee-**soh**-nah ehn ehl pah-**sah**-doh?

When was the last time you took Prednisone?

¿Cuándo fue la última vez que tomó Prednisona?
Kwahn-doh fweh lah **ool**-tee-mah behs keh toh-**moh** prehd-nee-**soh**-nah?

What do you think caused the attack?

¿Qué cree usted que causó el ataque?
Keh **kreh**-eh oos-**tehd** keh kah-oo-**soh** ehl ah-**tah**-keh?

The weather?

¿El clima?
Ehl **klee**-mah?

Dust?

¿Polvo?
Pohl-boh?

Exercise?

¿Ejercicio?
Eh-hehr-**see**-see-oh?

Cigarette smoke?

¿Humo de cigarrillo?
Oo-moh deh see-gah-**ree**-yoh?

Emotional upset?

¿Enojo emocional?
Eh-**noh**-hoh eh-moh-see-oh-**nahl**?

Something else?

¿Otra cosa?
Oh-trah **koh**-sah?

How many times a month do you have an asthma attack?	¿Cuántas veces al mes tiene un ataque de asma? **Kwahn**-tahs **beh**-sehs ahl mehs tee-**eh**-neh oon ah-**tah**-keh deh **ahs**-mah?
How many times have you been admitted in the past year for asthma?	¿Cuántas veces lo han internado por asma en el año pasado? **Kwahn**-tahs **beh**-sehs loh ahn een-tehr-**nah**-doh pohr **ahs**-mah ehn ehl **ah**-nyoh pah-**sah**-doh?
How many times have you been to the emergency room for an asthma attack in the past year?	¿Cuántas veces ha venido a la sala de emergencia por ataques de asma en el año pasado? **Kwahn**-tahs **beh**-sehs ah beh-**nee**-doh ah lah **sah**-lah deh eh-mehr-**hen**-see-ah pohr ah-**tah**-kehs deh **ahs**-mah ehn ehl **ah**-nyoh pah-**sah**-doh?
Have they admitted you to intensive care for asthma in the past?	¿Lo han internado en cuidado intensivo por asma en el pasado? Loh ahn een-tehr-**nah**-doh ehn kwi-**dah**-doh een-tehn-**see**-boh pohr oon ah-**tah**-keh deh **ahs**-mah ehn ehl pah-**sah**-doh?
Have you been intubated in the past for asthma?	¿Lo han intubado por asma en el pasado? Loh ahn een-too-**bah**-doh pohr **ahs**-mah ehn ehl pah-**sah**-doh?
Do you smoke?	¿Fuma usted? **Foo**-mah oos-**tehd**?

Was someone smoking next to you when the asthma attack started?

¿Alguien estaba fumando cerca de usted cuando empezó el ataque de asma?
Ahl-gee-ehn ehs-**tah**-bah foo-**mahn**-doh **sehr**-kah deh oos-**tehd kwahn**-doh ehm-peh-**soh** ehl ah-**tah**-keh deh **ahs**-mah?

Common Phrases for the Exam for Asthma

We are going to give you a treatment.

Vamos a darle un tratamiento.
Bah-mohs ah **dahr**-leh oon trah-tah-mee-**ehn**-toh.

You need an IV (intravenous line).

Usted necesita suero (línea intravenosa).
Oos-**tehd** neh-seh-**see**-tah soo-**eh**-roh (**lee**-neh-ah een-trah-beh-**noh**-sah).

We are going to give you medicine through the IV.

Le vamos a dar medicina por la línea intravenosa.
Leh **bah**-mohs ah dahr meh-dee-**see**-nah pohr lah **lee**-neh-ah een-trah-beh-**noh**-sah.

We need to take an X ray.

Es necesario sacarle una radiografía.
Ehs neh-seh-**sah**-ree-oh sah-**cahr**-leh **oo**-nah rah-dee-oh-grah-**fee**-ah.

I need to do an arterial blood test.

Necesito hacerle una prueba de sangre arterial.
Neh-seh-**see**-toh ah-**sehr**-leh **oo**-nah **prweh**-bah deh **sahn**-greh ahr-teh-ree-**ahl**.

We need to admit you.

Necesitamos internarlo / la.
Neh-seh-see-**tah**-mohs een-tehr-**nahr**-loh / -lah.

We need to intubate you.	Necesitamos intubarlo / la. Neh-seh-see-**tah**-mohs een-too-**bahr**-loh / -lah.
You have a pneumonia.	Usted tiene pulmonía. Oos-**tehd** tee-**eh**-neh pool-moh-**nee**-ah.

Discharge Instructions for Asthma

Take your medicine as indicated.	Tome su medicina como le indicaron. **Toh**-meh soo meh-dee-**see**-nah **koh**-moh leh een-dee-**kah**-rohn.
Return to the hospital (clinic) if you have . . .	Regrese al hospital (a la clínica) si tiene... Reh-**greh**-seh ahl ohs-pee-**tahl** (ah lah **klee**-nee-kah) see tee-**eh**-neh...
shortness of breath,	falta de aire, **fahl**-tah deh **ah**-ee-reh,
fever,	fiebre, fee-**eh**-breh,
or vomiting.	o vómito. oh **boh**-mee-toh.
Avoid cigarette smoke.	Evite el humo de cigarrillo. Eh-**bee**-teh ehl **oo**-moh deh see-gah-**ree**-yoh.

Abdominal/Genitourinary

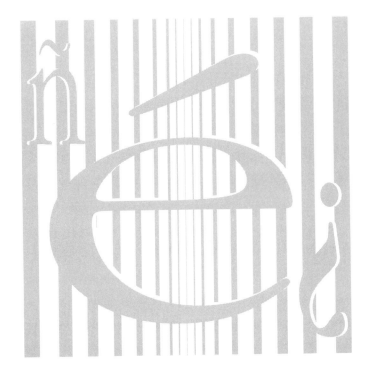

Abdominal Pain

Dolor Abdominal
Doh-**lohr** ab-doh-mee-nahl

Show me where the pain started.

Enséñeme dónde empezó el dolor.
Ehn-**seh**-nyeh-meh **dohn**-deh ehm-peh-**soh** ehl doh-**lohr**.

Show me with one finger where you have the pain.

Enséñeme con un solo dedo dónde tiene el dolor.
Ehn-**seh**-nyeh-meh kohn oon **soh**-loh **deh**-doh **dohn**-deh tee-**eh**-neh ehl doh-**lohr**.

For how many days or hours have you had pain?

¿Por cuántos días u horas ha tenido dolor?
Pohr **kwahn**-tohs **dee**-ahs oo **oh**-rahs ah teh-**nee**-doh doh-**lohr**?

Is the pain constant?

¿Es el dolor constante?
Ehs ehl doh-**lohr** kohns-**tahn**-teh?

Does the pain come and go?

¿El dolor le va y viene?
Ehl doh-**lohr** leh bah ee bee-**eh**-neh?

Does the pain go to the back?

¿Le viaja el dolor a la espalda?
Leh bee-**ah**-ha ehl doh-**lohr** ah lah ehs-**pahl**-dah?

Does the pain go to the testicles?

¿Le viaja el dolor a los testículos?
Leh bee-**ah**-ha ehl doh-**lohr** ah lohs tehs-**tee**-koo-lohs?

Does the pain go to the groin?

¿Le viaja el dolor a la ingle?
Leh bee-**ah**-ha ehl doh-**lohr** ah lah **een**-gleh?

Does the pain go to the bladder?

¿Le viaja el dolor a la vejiga?
Leh bee-**ah**-ha ehl doh-**lohr** ah lah beh-**hee**-gah?

Have you gotten worse since the pain started?

¿Ha empeorado desde que comenzó el dolor?
Ah ehm-peh-oh-**rah**-doh **dehs**-deh keh koh-mehn-**soh** ehl doh-**lohr**?

Do you have nausea?

¿Tiene náusea?
Tee-**eh**-neh **nah**-oo-seh-ah?

Do you have vomiting?

¿Tiene vómito?
Tee-**eh**-neh **boh**-mee-toh?

Did the pain or the vomiting start first?

¿Empezó primero el dolor o el vómito?
Ehm-peh-**soh** pree-**meh**-roh ehl doh-**lohr** oh ehl **boh**-mee-toh?

How many times have you vomited today?

¿Cuántas veces ha vomitado hoy?
Kwahn-tahs **beh**-sehs ah boh-mee-**tah**-doh **oh**-ee?

When was the last time that you vomited?

¿Cuándo fue la última vez que vomitó?
Kwahn-doh **fweh** lah **ool**-tee-mah behs keh boh-mee-**toh**?

(X) hours (days) ago.

(X) horas (días).
(X) **oh**-rahs (**dee**-ahs).

Have you been able to retain any water or food since you last vomited?

¿Ha podido retener agua o comida desde la última vez que vomitó?
Ah poh-**dee**-doh reh-teh-**nehr** **ah**-gwah oh koh-**mee**-dah **dehs**-deh lah **ool**-tee-mah behs keh boh-mee-**toh**?

When was the last time that you ate?	¿Cuándo fue la última vez que comió? **Kwahn**-doh **fweh** lah **ool**-tee-mah behs **keh koh**-mee-oh?
(X) hours ago.	(X) horas. (X) **oh**-rahs.
Do you have diarrhea?	¿Tiene diarrea? Tee-**eh**-neh dee-ah-**rhe**-ah?
How many times today?	¿Cuántas veces hoy? **Kwahn**-tahs **beh**-sehs oh-ee?
Are you constipated?	¿Está estreñido / -a? Ehs-**tah** ehs-treh-**nyee**-doh / -dah?
Are you passing gas?	¿Está pasando gas? Ehs-**tah** pah-**sahn**-doh gahs?
Have they told you if you have . . .	Le han dicho si tiene... Leh ahn **dee**-choh see tee-**eh**-neh...
gastritis?	gastritis? gahs-**tree**-tees?
pancreatitis?	pancreatitis? pahn-kreh-ah-**tee**-tees?
stomach ulcers?	úlceras en el estómago? **ool**-seh-rahs ehn ehl ehs-**toh**-mah-goh?
hepatitis?	hepatitis? eh-pah-**tee**-tees?
colitis?	colitis? koh-**lee**-tees?

kidney stones?

cálculos o piedras en el riñón?
kahl-koo-lohs oh pee-**eh**-drahs ehn ehl ree-**nyohn**?

gallstones?

cálculos o piedras en la vesícula?
kahl-koo-lohs oh pee-**eh**-drahs ehn lah beh-**see**-koo-lah?

Does it burn when you urinate?

¿Le arde cuando orina?
Leh **ahr**-deh **kwahn**-doh oh-**ree**-nah?

Are you urinating frequently?

¿Está orinando frecuentemente?
Ehs-**tah** oh-ree-**nahn**-doh freh-kwehn-teh-**mehn**-teh?

Have you noticed blood in your urine?

¿Ha notado sangre en la orina?
Ah noh-**tah**-doh **sahn**-greh ehn lah oh-**ree**-nah?

What color is your urine?

¿De qué color es su orina?
Deh keh koh-**lohr** ehs soo oh-**ree**-nah?

Is it yellow?

¿Es amarilla?
Ehs ah-mah-**ree**-yah?

Is it red?

¿Es roja?
Ehs **roh**-hah?

Is it brown?

¿Es color café?
Ehs koh-**lohr** kah-**feh**?

Have you had any abdominal surgery?

¿Ha tenido alguna operación abdominal?
Ah teh-**nee**-doh ahl-**goo**-nah oh-peh-rah-see-**ohn** ab-doh-mee-**nahl**?

Do you drink alcohol?

¿Toma bebidas alcohólicas?
Toh-mah beh-**bee**-dahs ahl-**koh**-lee-kahs?

When was your last drink?

¿Cuándo tomó su última bebida alcohólica?
Kwahn-doh toh-**moh** soo **ool**-tee-mah beh-**bee**-dah ahl-**koh**-lee-kah?

Common Phrases for the Exam for Abdominal Pain

I need to do a rectal exam.

Necesito hacerle un examen del recto.
Neh-seh-**see**-toh ah-**sehr**-leh oon ek-**sah**-mehn dehl **rek**-toh.

I need to do a genital exam.

Necesito hacerle un examen genital.
Neh-seh-**see**-toh ah-**sehr**-leh oon ek-**sah**-mehn he-nee-**tahl**.

I need to do a pelvic exam.

Necesito hacerle un examen pélvico.
Neh-seh-**see**-toh ah-**sehr**-leh oon ek-**sah**-mehn **pehl**-bee-koh.

I am going to examine your abdomen.

Voy a examinarle el abdomen.
Boy ah ek-sah-mee-**nahr**-leh ehl ab-**doh**-mehn.

Bend your knees.

Doble las rodillas.
Doh-bleh lahs roh-**dee**-yahs.

Do you have pain here?

¿Tiene dolor aquí?
Tee-**eh**-neh doh-**lohr** ah-**kee**?

Do you have pain when I hit (palpate / touch) your back?	¿Tiene dolor cuando le pego (palpo / toco) en la espalda? Tee-**eh**-neh doh-**lohr kwahn**-doh leh **peh**-goh (**pahl**-poh / **toh**-koh) ehn lah ehs-**pahl**-dah?
We need to do blood and urine tests.	Necesitamos hacerle pruebas de sangre y orina. Neh-seh-see-**tah**-mohs ah-**sehr**-leh **prweh**-bahs deh **sahn**-greh ee oh-**ree**-nah.
We are going to take some X rays.	Vamos a sacarle unas radiografías. **Bah**-mohs ah sah-**kahr**-leh **oo**-nahs rah-dee-oh-grah-**fee**-ahs.
You need an ultrasound.	Usted necesita un ultrasonido. Oos-**tehd** neh-seh-**see**-tah oon ool-trah-soh-**nee**-doh.
You need an operation.	Usted necesita una operación. Oos-**tehd** neh-seh-**see**-tah **oo**-nah oh-peh-rah-see-**ohn**.
You have gallstones.	Tiene piedras en la vesícula. Tee-**eh**-neh pee-**eh**-drahs ehn lah beh-**see**-koo-lah.
You have appendicitis.	Tiene apendicitis. Tee-**eh**-neh ah-pehn-dee-**see**-tees.
You have inflammation of the pancreas.	Tiene inflamación del páncreas. Tee-**eh**-neh een-flah-mah-see-**ohn** dehl **pahn**-kreh-ahs.
You have a stomach ulcer.	Tiene úlcera en el estómago. Tee-**eh**-neh **ool**-seh-rah ehn ehl ehs-**toh**-mah-goh.

You have gastritis.	Tiene gastritis. Tee-**eh**-neh gahs-**tree**-tees.

Discharge Instructions for Abdominal Pain

Return to the hospital (clinic) if . . .	Regrese al hospital (a la clínica) si... Reh-**greh**-seh ahl ohs-pee-**tahl** (ah lah **klee**-nee-kah) see...
you have a fever,	tiene fiebre, tee-**eh**-neh fee-**eh**-breh,
you have vomiting,	tiene vómito, tee-**eh**-neh **boh**-mee-toh,
the pain is worse or increases,	el dolor se pone peor o aumenta, ehl doh-**lohr** seh **poh**-neh peh-**ohr** oh ah-oo-**mehn**-tah,
or you are unable to retain fluids or food.	o si no puede retener líquidos o comida. oh see noh **pweh**-deh reh-teh-**nehr lee**-kee-dohs oh koh-**mee**-dah.

Nausea and Vomiting

Náusea y Vómito

Nah-oo-seh-ah ee **boh**-mee-toh

How many times a day have you been vomiting?	¿Cuántas veces vomita por día? **Kwahn**-tahs **beh**-sehs boh-**mee**-tah pohr **dee**-ah?

How many days have you had vomiting?	¿Por cuántos días ha tenido vómito? Pohr **kwahn**-tohs **dee**-ahs ah teh-**nee**-doh **boh**-mee-toh?
Have you vomited liquids (food, fresh blood)?	¿Ha vomitado usted líquidos (comida, sangre fresca)? A boh-mee-**tah**-doh oos-**tehd lee**-kee-dohs (koh-**mee**-dah, **sahn**-greh **frehs**-kah)?
What color is the vomit?	¿De qué color es el vómito? Deh keh koh-**lohr** ehs ehl **boh**-mee-toh?
Do you have nausea?	¿Tiene náusea? Tee-**eh**-neh **nah**-oo-seh-ah?
Do you have diarrhea?	¿Tiene diarrea? Tee-**eh**-neh dee-ah-**reh**-ah?
Since when?	¿Desde cuándo? **Dehs**-deh **kwahn**-doh?
How many times a day do you have diarrhea?	¿Cuántas veces al día tiene diarrea? **Kwahn**-tahs **beh**-sehs ahl **dee**-ah tee-**eh**-neh dee-ah-**reh**-ah?
Do you have blood in your stool?	¿Ha notado sangre en el excremento o heces? Ah noh-**tah**-doh **sahn**-greh ehn ehl eks-kreh-**mehn**-toh oh **eh**-sehs?
What color is your stool?	¿De qué color son sus heces? Deh keh koh-**lohr** sohn soos **eh**-sehs? *or* ¿De qué color es su excremento? Deh keh koh-**lohr** ehs soo eks-kreh-**mehn**-toh?

Do you have pain in your abdomen?

¿Tiene usted dolor en el abdomen / vientre?
Tee-**eh**-neh oos-**tehd** doh-**lohr** ehn ehl ab-**doh**-mehn / **biehn**-treh?

Does your pain go away when you use the bathroom?

¿Se le quita el dolor cuando usa el baño?
Seh leh **kee**-tah ehl doh-**lohr** **kwahn**-doh **oo**-sah ehl **bah**-nyoh?

Have you had fever?

¿Ha tenido fiebre?
Ah teh-**nee**-doh fee-**eh**-breh?

Do you have dizziness?

¿Tiene mareos?
Tee-**eh**-neh mah-**reh**-ohs?

Have you traveled recently to another state or country?

¿Ha viajado recientemente a otro estado o país?
Ah bee-ah-**hah**-doh reh-see-ehn-teh-**mehn**-teh ah **oh**-troh ehs-**tah**-doh o pah-**ees**?

Did you eat something that made you sick?

¿Comió algo que le haya hecho daño?
Koh-mee-**oh ahl**-goh keh leh **ah**-yah **eh**-choh **dah**-nyoh?

Do you vomit when you eat greasy or fried food?

¿Vomita cuando come comidas grasosas o fritas?
Boh-**mee**-tah **kwahn**-doh koh-meh koh-**mee**-dahs grah-**soh**-sahs oh **free**-tahs?

Is there anyone else in your family who is ill with vomiting or diarrhea?

¿Alguien más en su familia ha estado enfermo con vómito o diarrea?
Ahl-gee-ehn mahs ehn soo fah-**mee**-lee-ah ah ehs-**tah**-doh ehn-**fehr**-moh kohn **boh**-mee-toh oh dee-ah-**reh**-ah?

Today have you been able to retain food or water in your stomach?

¿Hoy ha podido retener comida o agua en el estómago?

Oh-ee ah poh-**dee**-doh reh-teh-**nehr** koh-**mee**-dah oh **ah**-gwah ehn ehl ehs-**toh**-mah-goh?

Do you have a cold or the flu?

¿Tiene gripe o catarro?

Tee-**eh**-neh **gree**-peh oh kah-**tah**-roh?

Do you get stomach pains before the diarrhea?

¿Le dan dolores del estómago antes de la diarrea?

Leh dahn doh-**loh**-rehs dehl ehs-**toh**-mah-goh **ahn**-tehs deh lah dee-ah-**reh**-ah?

Have you had parasites or amebas?

¿Ha tenido parásitos o amebas?

Ah teh-**nee**-doh pah-**rah**-see-tohs oh ah-**meh**-bahs?

Do you suffer from a . . .

Padece usted de...

Pah-**deh**-seh oos-**tehd** deh...

stomach ulcer?

úlcera del estómago?

ool-seh-rah dehl ehs-**toh**-mah-goh?

gallstone?

cálculo en la vesícula?

kahl-koo-loh ehn lah beh-**see**-koo-lah?

kidney stone?

cálculo en el riñón?

kahl-koo-loh ehn ehl ree-**nyohn**?

Have you been in contact with someone who has hepatitis?

¿Ha estado en contacto con alguien que tenga hepatitis?

Ah ehs-**tah**-doh ehn kohn-**tak**-toh kohn **ahl**-gee-ehn keh **tehn**-gah eh-pah-**tee**-tees?

Common Phrases for the Exam for Nausea and Vomiting

Show me where the pain is.

Enséñeme dónde tiene el dolor.

Ehn-**seh**-nyeh-meh **dohn**-deh tee-**eh**-neh ehl doh-**lohr**.

I need to examine your abdomen.

Necesito examinarle el abdomen.

Neh-seh-**see**-toh ek-sah-mee-**nahr**-leh ehl ab-**doh**-mehn.

Bend your knees.

Doble las rodillas.

Doh-bleh lahs roh-**dee**-yahs.

Breathe deeply.

Respire profundo.

Rehs-**pee**-reh proh-**foon**-doh.

I need to do a rectal exam.

Necesito hacerle un examen del recto.

Neh-seh-**see**-toh ah-**sehr**-leh oon ek-**sah**-mehn dehl **rek**-toh.

I need to do blood and urine tests.

Necesito hacerle análisis de sangre y orina.

Neh-seh-**see**-toh ah-**sehr**-leh ah-**nah**-lee-sees deh **sahn**-greh ee oh-**ree**-nah.

You need an IV.

Usted necesita suero intravenoso.

Oos-**tehd** neh-seh-**see**-tah soo-**eh**-roh een-trah-beh-**noh**-soh.

We need to take an X ray of your abdomen.

Es necesario sacarle radiografías de su abdomen.

Ehs neh-seh-**sah**-ree-oh sah-**kahr**-leh rah-dee-oh-grah-**fee**-ahs deh soo ab-**doh**-mehn.

Discharge Instructions for Nausea and Vomiting

Return to the hospital (clinic) if . . .

Regrese al hospital (a la clínica) si...
Reh-**greh**-seh ahl ohs-pee-**tahl** (ah lah **klee**-nee-kah) see...

you are vomiting blood, have fever or dizziness,

vomita sangre, tiene fiebre o mareos,
boh-**mee**-tah **sahn**-greh, tee-**eh**-neh fee-**eh**-breh oh mah-**reh**-ohs,

you continue vomiting,

sigue vomitando,
see-geh boh-mee-**tahn**-doh,

or you see blood in your stool.

o nota sangre en el excremento (las heces).
oh **noh**-tah **sahn**-greh ehn ehl eks-kreh-**mehn**-toh (lahs **eh**-sehs).

Avoid greasy foods, spicy foods, and alcohol.

Evite comidas grasosas o picantes, y las bebidas alcohólicas.
Eh-**bee**-teh koh-**mee**-dahs grah-**soh**-sahs oh pee-**kahn**-tehs, ee lahs beh-**bee**-dahs ahl-**koh**-lee-kahs.

Drink clear liquids, such as broth, Jell-O, soft drinks, and juice.

Tome líquidos claros como consomé, gelatina, refrescos, y jugo.
Toh-meh **lee**-kee-dohs **klah**-rohs **koh**-moh kohn-soh-**meh**, he-lah-**tee**-nah, reh-**frehs**-kohs, ee **hoo**-go.

Diarrhea

Diarrea
Dee-ah-**reh**-ah

How many days have you had diarrhea?

¿Por cuántos días ha tenido diarrea?
Pohr **kwahn**-tohs **dee**-ahs ah teh-**nee**-doh dee-ah-**reh**-ah?

How many times have you had diarrhea today?

¿Cuántas veces ha tenido diarrea hoy?
Kwahn-tahs **beh**-sehs ah teh-**nee**-doh dee-ah-**reh**-ah **oo**-ee?

What color is the diarrhea?

¿De qué color es la diarrea?
Deh keh koh-**lohr** ehs lah dee-ah-**reh**-ah?

Is it yellow?

¿Es amarilla?
Ehs ah-mah-**ree**-yah?

Is it green?

¿Es verde?
Ehs **behr**-deh?

Is it black?

¿Es negra?
Ehs **neh**-grah?

Have you noticed blood in the diarrhea?

¿Ha notado sangre en la diarrea?
Ah noh-**tah**-doh **sahn**-greh ehn lah dee-ah-**reh**-ah?

Do you have abdominal pain?

¿Tiene dolor abdominal?
Tee-**eh**-neh doh-**lohr** ab-doh-mee-**nahl**?

What is the pain like?

¿Cómo es el dolor?
Koh-moh ehs ehl doh-**lohr**?

Is it acute / sharp?	¿Es agudo? Ehs ah-**goo**-doh?
Is it piercing?	¿Es punzante? Ehs poon-**sahn**-teh?
Does it burn?	¿Es quemante? Ehs keh-**mahn**-teh?
Is it like cramps?	¿Es como calambres / cólico? Ehs **koh**-moh kah-**lahm**-brehs / **koh**-lee-koh?
Is it like a pressure?	¿Es opresivo? Ehs oh-preh-**see**-boh?
Does the pain go away after you have diarrhea?	¿Se le quita el dolor después de tener diarrea? Seh leh **kee**-tah ehl doh-**lohr** dehs-**pwehs** deh teh-**nehr** dee-ah-**reh**-ah?
Do you have a fever?	¿Tiene fiebre? Tee-**eh**-neh fee-**eh**-breh?
Do you have nausea or vomiting?	¿Tiene náusea o vómito? Tee-**eh**-neh **nah**-oo-seh-ah oh **boh**-mee-toh?
Do you have dizziness?	¿Tiene mareos? Tee-**eh**-neh mah-**reh**-ohs?
Have you recently traveled outside the country or state?	¿Ha viajado recientemente fuera del país o del estado? Ah bee-ah-**ha**-doh reh-see-ehn-teh-**mehn**-teh **fweh**-rah dehl pah-**ees** oh dehl ehs-**tah**-doh?

Have you eaten in fast-food restaurants recently?	¿Ha comido en restaurantes de comida rápida (como McDonald's) recientemente? Ah koh-**mee**-doh ehn rehs-tah-oo-**rahn**-tehs deh koh-**mee**-dah **rah**-pee-dah (**koh**-moh Mahk-**Doh**-nahlds) reh-see-ehn-teh-**mehn**-teh?
Is there someone living with you who has the same symptoms?	¿Hay alguien que vive con usted que tenga los mismos síntomas? **Ah**-ee **ahl**-gee-ehn keh **bee**-beh kohn oos-**tehd** keh **tehn**-gah lohs **mees**-mohs **seen**-toh-mahs?
Do you have diabetes?	¿Tiene diabetes? Tee-**eh**-neh dee-ah-**beh**-tehs?
Normally, how many bowel movements do you have a day?	Normalmente, ¿cuántas veces va al baño (obra) al día? Nohr-mahl-**mehn**-teh, **kwahn**-tahs **beh**-sehs bah ahl **bah**-nyoh ahl **dee**-ah? *or* Nohr-mahl-**mehn**-teh, **kwahn**-tahs **beh**-sehs **oh**-brah ahl **dee**-ah?

Common Phrases for the Exam for Diarrhea

I need to do a rectal exam.	Necesito hacerle un examen del recto. Neh-seh-**see**-toh ah-**sehr**-leh oon ek-**sah**-mehn dehl **rek**-toh.
Can you give us a stool sample?	¿Puede darnos una muestra de excremento? **Pweh**-deh **dahr**-nohs **oo**-nah **mwehs**-trah deh eks-kreh-**mehn**-toh?

You need antibiotics.	Usted necesita antibióticos. Oos-**tehd** neh-seh-**see**-tah ahn-tee-bee-**oh**-tee-kohs.
You have a viral infection; you don't need antibiotics.	Usted tiene una infección viral; no necesita antibióticos. Oos-**tehd** tee-**eh**-neh **oo**-nah een-fek-see-**ohn** bee-**rahl**; noh neh-seh-**see**-tah ahn-tee-bee-**oh**-tee-kohs.

Discharge Instructions for Diarrhea

Return to the hospital (clinic) if . . .	Regrese al hospital (a la clínica) si... Reh-**greh**-seh ahl ohs-pee-**tahl** (ah lah **klee**-nee-kah) see...
you have fever,	tiene fiebre, tee-**eh**-neh fee-**eh**-breh,
you have vomiting,	tiene vómito, tee-**eh**-neh **boh**-mee-toh,
you have blood in your stools,	tiene sangre en sus heces o excremento, tee-**eh**-neh **sahn**-greh ehn soos **eh**-sehs oh eks-kreh-**mehn**-toh,
or the abdominal pain gets worse.	o el dolor abdominal es peor. oh ehl doh-**lohr** ab-doh-mee-**nahl** ehs peh-**ohr**.

Constipation

When was the last time you had a bowel movement?

Normally do you have a bowel movement every day?

Every how many days do you have a bowel movement now?

Have you noticed if your stools are thinner (harder)?

Have you noticed blood mixed with the stools?

Have you noticed blood only when you wipe?

Estreñimiento

Ehs-treh-nyee-mee-**ehn**-toh

¿Cuándo fue la última vez que obró (que usó el baño)?
Kwahn-doh fweh lah **ool**-tee-mah behs keh oh-**broh** (keh oo-**soh** ehl **bah**-nyoh)?

¿Normalmente obra usted todos los días?
Nohr-mahl-**mehn**-teh **oh**-brah oos-**tehd toh**-dohs lohs **dee**-ahs?

¿Cada cuantos días obra ahora?
Kah-dah **kwahn**-tohs **dee**-ahs **oh**-brah ah-**oh**-rah?

¿Ha notado que sus heces son mas delgadas (duras)?
Ah noh-**tah**-doh keh soos **eh**-sehs sohn mahs dehl-**gah**-dahs (**doo**-rahs)?

¿Ha notado sangre mezclada con sus heces?
Ah noh-**tah**-doh **sahn**-greh mehs-**klah**-dah kohn soos **eh**-sehs?

¿Ha notado sangre solamente cuando se limpia?
Ah noh-**tah**-doh **sahn**-greh soh-lah-**mehn**-teh **kwahn**-doh seh **leem**-pee-ah?

What color are your stools?	¿De qué color son sus heces? Deh keh koh-**lohr** sohn soos **eh**-sehs?
Are they yellow?	¿Son amarillas? Sohn ah-mah-**ree**-yahs?
Are they brown?	¿Son de color café? Sohn deh koh-**lohr** kah-**feh**?
Are they green?	¿Son verdes? Sohn **behr**-dehs?
Are they black?	¿Son negras? Sohn **neh**-grahs?
Have you had diarrhea before becoming constipated?	¿Ha tenido diarrea antes de estreñirse? Ah teh-**nee**-doh dee-ah-**reh**-ah **ahn**-tehs deh ehs-treh-**nyeer**-seh?
Do you frequently use laxatives?	¿Usa laxantes frecuentemente? **Oo**-sah lak-**sahn**-tehs freh-kwehn-teh-**mehn**-teh?
Do you have abdominal pain?	¿Tiene dolor en el abdomen? Tee-**eh**-neh doh-**lohr** ehn ehl ab-**doh**-mehn?
Do you have nausea or vomiting?	¿Tiene náusea o vómito? Tee-**eh**-neh **nah**-oo-seh-ah oh **boh**-mee-toh?
Do you have a fever?	¿Tiene fiebre? Tee-**eh**-neh fee-**eh**-breh?

Common Phrases for the Exam for Constipation

I need to do a rectal exam.

Necesito hacerle un examen del recto.
Neh-seh-**see**-toh ah-**sehr**-leh oon ek-**sah**-mehn dehl **rek**-toh.

You have a fecal impaction.

Usted está tapado / -a con heces.
Oos-**tehd** ehs-**tah** tah-**pah**-doh / -dah kohn **eh**-sehs.

We need to give you an enema.

Necesitamos darle una enema.
Neh-seh-see-**tah**-mohs **dahr**-leh **oo**-nah eh-**neh**-mah.

Discharge Instructions for Constipation

Eat a lot of fresh fruit and vegetables.

Coma muchas verduras y frutas frescas.
Koh-mah **moo**-chahs behr-**doo**-rahs ee **froo**-tahs **frehs**-kahs.

Drink eight glasses of water a day.

Tome ocho vasos de agua al día.
Toh-meh **oh**-choh **bah**-sohs deh **ah**-gwah ahl **dee**-ah.

Do not use laxatives.

No use laxantes.
Noh **oo**-seh lak-**sahn**-tehs.

You can take Metamucil.

Puede tomar Metamucil.
Pweh-deh toh-**mahr** Meh-tah-moo-**seel**.

Jaundice

Ictericia
Eek-teh-**ree**-see-ah

How long has your skin been yellow?	¿Desde cuándo tiene la piel amarilla? **Dehs**-deh **kwahn**-doh tee-**eh**-neh lah pee-**ehl** ah-mah-**ree**-yah?
Do you have abdominal pain?	¿Tiene dolor abdominal? Tee-**eh**-neh doh-**lohr** abh-doh-mee-**nahl**?
Do you have nausea or vomiting?	¿Tiene náusea o vómito? Tee-**eh**-neh **nah**-oo-seh-ah oh **boh**-mee-toh?
What color is your urine?	¿De qué color es su orina? Deh keh koh-**lohr** ehs soo oh-**ree**-nah?
Is it clear yellow?	¿Es amarilla clara? Ehs ah-mah-**ree**-yah **klah**-rah?
Is it dark yellow?	¿Es amarilla obscura? Ehs ah-mah-**ree**-yah ohbs-**koo**-rah?
Is it Coca-cola color?	¿Es el color de Coca-cola? Ehs ehl koh-**lohr** deh **koh**-kah **koh**-lah?
What color are your stools?	¿De qué color son sus heces? Deh keh koh-**lohr** sohn soos **eh**-sehs?
Are they yellow?	¿Son amarillas? Sohn ah-mah-**ree**-yahs?

Are they brown?	¿Son de color café? Sohn deh koh-**lohr** kah-**feh**?
Are they black?	¿Son negras? Sohn **neh**-grahs?
Do your stools float in the toilet bowl?	¿Sus heces flotan en la taza del inodoro / retrete? Soos **eh**-sehs **floh**-tahn ehn lah **tah**-sah dehl ee-noh-**doh**-roh / reh-**treh**-teh?
Have you recently had contact with a person with hepatitis?	¿Ha tenido contacto recientemente con una persona con hepatitis? Ah teh-**nee**-doh kohn-**tahk**-toh reh-see-ehn-teh-**mehn**-teh kohn **oo**-nah pehr-**soh**-nah kohn eh-pah-**tee**-tees?
Do you have a fever?	¿Tiene fiebre? Tee-**eh**-neh fee-**eh**-breh?
If you smoke, does the taste of the cigarette bother you?	Si usted fuma, ¿le molesta el sabor del cigarrillo? See oos-**tehd foo**-mah, leh moh-**lehs**-tah ehl sah-**bohr** dehl see-gah-**ree**-yoh?
Do you drink alcohol?	¿Toma usted bebidas alcohólicas? **Toh**-mah oos-**tehd** beh-**bee**-dahs ahl-**koh**-lee-kahs?
Did you leave the country recently?	¿Salió del país recientemente? Sah-lee-**oh** dehl pah-**ees** reh-see-ehn-teh-**mehn**-teh?
Where did you go?	¿A dónde fue? Ah **dohn**-deh foo-**eh**?

Mexico?	¿A México? Ah **Meh**-hee-koh?
India?	¿A la India? Ah lah Een-dee-ah?
The Far East?	¿A un país asiático? Ah oon pah-**ees** ah- see-**ah**-tee-koh?
Africa?	¿A África? Ah **Ah**-free-kah?
Central or South America?	¿A la América Central o América del Sur? Ah lah Ah-**meh**-ree- kah Sehn-**trahl** oh Ah-**meh**-ree-kah dehl soor?
Have you received the hepatitis vaccine?	¿Ha recibido la vacuna de hepatitis? Ah reh-see-**bee**-doh lah bah- **koo**-nah deh eh-pah-**tee**-tees?
Have you received a blood transfusion recently?	¿Ha recibido una transfusión de sangre recientemente? Ah reh-see-**bee**-doh **oo**-nah trahns-foo-see-**ohn** deh **sahn**- greh reh-see-ehn-teh-**mehn**- teh?
Do you have any liver diseases?	¿Sufre usted de enfermedades del hígado? **Soo**-freh oos-**tehd** deh ehn- fehr-meh-**dah**-dehs dehl **ee**- gah-doh?
Do you have . . .	¿Sufre de... **Soo**-freh deh...
hepatitis?	hepatitis? eh-pah-**tee**-tees?

cirrhosis of the liver?	cirrhosis? see-**roh**-sees?
gallstones?	piedras en la vesícula? pee-**eh**-drahs ehn lah beh-**see**-koo-lah?
pancreatitis?	pancreatitis? pahn-kreh-ah-**tee**-tees?
Do you have sexual relations with men (women, prostitutes)?	¿Tiene usted relaciones sexuales con hombres (mujeres, prostitutas)? Tee-**eh**-neh oos-**tehd** reh-lah-see-**oh**-nehs sek-soo-**ah**-lehs kohn **ohm**-brehs (moo-**heh**-rehs, prohs-tee-**too**-tahs)?
Do you take medicine?	¿Toma usted medicina? **Toh**-mah oos-**tehd** meh-dee-**see**-nah?
What type?	¿De qué tipo? Deh keh **tee**-poh?
Do you have the medicine with you?	¿Trae la medicina con usted? **Trah**-eh lah meh-dee-**see**-nah kohn oos-**tehd**?
When was the last time you took the medicine?	¿Cuándo fue la última vez que tomó la medicina? **Kwahn**-doh fweh lah **ool**-tee-mah behs keh toh-**moh** lah meh-dee-**see**-nah?
(X) hours (days, weeks) ago.	(X) horas (días, semanas). (X) **oh**-rahs (**dee**-ahs, seh-**mah**-nahs).

Do you have problems with your blood clotting?	¿Tiene problemas con la coagulación de la sangre? Tee-**eh**-neh proh-**bleh**-mahs kohn lah koh-ah-goo-lah-see-**ohn** deh lah **sahn**-greh?
Do you frequently eat at fast-food restaurants?	¿Usted come frecuentemente en restaurantes de comida rápida? Oos-**tehd koh**-meh freh-kwehn-teh-**mehn**-teh ehn rehs-tah-oo-**rahn**-tehs deh koh-**mee**-dah **rah**-pee-dah?
Do you work in a restaurant?	¿Trabaja usted en un restaurante? Trah-**bah**-hah oos-**tehd** ehn oon rehs-tah-oo-**rahn**-teh?
Do you prepare the food?	¿Prepara usted la comida? Preh-**pah**-rah oos-**tehd** lah koh-**mee**-dah?

Common Phrases for the Exam for Jaundice

We are going to do blood and urine tests.	Vamos a hacerle pruebas de orina y sangre. **Bah**-mohs ah ah-**sehr**-leh **prweh**-bahs deh oh-**ree**-nah ee **sahn**-greh.
We are going to do a hepatitis test.	Vamos a hacerle una prueba de hepatitis. **Bah**-mohs ah ah-**sehr**-leh **oo**-nah **prweh**-bah deh eh-pah-**tee**-tees.
We are going to do an ultrasound of the liver and gallbladder.	Vamos a hacerle un ultrasonido del hígado y la vesícula. **Bah**-mohs ah ah-**sehr**-leh oon ool-trah-soh-**nee**-doh dehl **ee**-gah-doh ee lah beh-**see**-koo-lah.

We are going to admit you.	Vamos a internarlo / -la.
	Bah-mohs ah een-tehr-**nahr**-loh / -lah.

Discharge Instructions for Jaundice

Return to the hospital (clinic) if . . .	Regrese al hospital (a la clínica) si...
	Reh-**greh**-seh ahl ohs-pee-**tahl** (ah lah **klee**-nee-kah) see...
you have constant abdominal pain,	tiene dolor abdominal constante,
	tee-**eh**-neh doh-**lohr** ab-doh-mee-**nahl** kohns-**tahn**-teh,
you have persistent vomiting,	tiene vómito persistente,
	tee-**eh**-neh **boh**-mee-toh pehr-sis-**tehn**-teh,
you have fever,	tiene fiebre,
	tee-**eh**-neh fee-**eh**-breh,
or you start bleeding.	o si usted empieza a sangrar.
	oh see oos-**tehd** ehm-pee-**eh**-sah ah sahn-**grahr**.
Don't have sex.	No tenga relaciones sexuales.
	Noh **tehn**-gah reh-lah-see-**oh**-nehs sek-soo-**ah**-lehs.
See your doctor for the results of the blood test.	Consulte con su doctor para los resultados de las pruebas de sangre.
	Kohn-**sool**-teh kohn soo dohk-**tohr pah**-rah lohs reh-sool-**tah**-dohs deh lahs **prweh**-bahs deh **sahn**-greh.

Upper Gastrointestinal (UGI) Bleeding

Sangrado Gastrointestinal Alto

Sahn-**grah**-doh gahs-troh-een-tehs-tee-nahl ahl-toh

How many times have you vomited today?

¿Cuántas veces ha vomitado hoy?
Kwahn-tahs **beh**-sehs ah boh-mee-**tah**-doh **oh**-ee?

What color is the blood that you vomited?

¿De qué color es la sangre que vomitó?
Deh keh koh-**lohr** ehs lah **sahn**-greh keh boh-mee-**toh**?

Is it the color of fresh blood?

¿Es del color de sangre fresca?
Ehs dehl koh-**lohr** deh **sahn**-greh **frehs**-kah?

Is it brown?

¿Es de color café?
Ehs deh koh-**lohr** kah-**feh**?

Is it black?

¿Es negra?
Ehs **neh**-grah?

When did the bleeding start?

¿Cuándo empezó el sangrado?
Kwahn-doh ehm-peh-**soh** ehl sahn-**grah**-doh?

Do you have abdominal pain?

¿Tiene dolor abdominal?
Tee-**eh**-neh doh-**lohr** ab-doh-mee-**nahl**?

Have you noticed blood in your stool?

¿Ha notado sangre en sus heces?
Ah noh-**tah**-doh **sahn**-greh ehn soos **eh**-sehs?

What color are your stools?	¿De qué color son sus heces? Deh keh koh-**lohr** sohn soos **eh**-sehs?
Are they yellow?	¿Son amarillas? Sohn ah-mah-**ree**-yahs?
Are they brown?	¿Son de color café? Sohn deh koh-**lohr** kah-**feh**?
Are they black?	¿Son negras? Sohn **neh**-grahs?
Do you have stomach ulcers?	¿Tiene úlceras del estómago? Tee-**eh**-neh **ool**-seh-rahs dehl ehs-**toh**-mah-goh?
Do you take medicine for the ulcers?	¿Toma medicina para las úlceras? **Toh**-mah meh-dee-**see**-nah **pah**-rah lahs **ool**-seh-rahs?
Do you take . . .	¿Toma... **Toh**-mah...
Zantac?	Zantac? **Sahn**-tak?
Tagamet?	Tagamet? Tah-gah-**meht**?
Pepcid?	Pepcid? Pep-**seed**?
Mylanta or Maalox?	Mylanta o Maalox? Mee-**lahn**-tah oh **Mah**-loks?
a different medicine?	otra medicina? **oh**-trah meh-dee-**see**-nah?

Do you . . .	¿Toma usted... **Toh**-mah oos-**tehd**...
take aspirin?	aspirinas? ahs-pee-**ree**-nahs?
take Motrin or ibuprofen?	Motrin o ibuprofen? **Moh**-treen oh ee-boo-**proh**-fehn?
drink alcohol?	bebidas alcohólicas? beh-**bee**-das ahl-**koh**-lee-kahs?
Do you have chest pain?	¿Tiene dolor del pecho? Tee-**eh**-neh doh-**lohr** dehl **peh**-choh?
Do you feel dizzy?	¿Se siente mareado / -a? Seh see-**ehn**-teh mah-reh-**ah**-doh / -dah?
Have you had bleeding from your stomach in the past?	¿Ha tenido sangrado del estómago en el pasado? Ah teh-**nee**-doh sahn-**grah**-doh dehl ehs-**toh**-mah-goh ehn ehl pah-**sah**-doh?
Have you had surgery for the ulcers?	¿Ha tenido cirugía para las úlceras? Ah teh-**nee**-doh see-roo-**hee**-ah **pah**-rah lahs **ool**-seh-rahs?
Do you have problems with your blood clotting?	¿Tiene usted problemas con la coagulación de la sangre? Tee-**eh**-neh oos-**tehd** proh-**bleh**-mahs kohn lah koh-ah-goo-lah-see-**ohn** deh lah **sahn**-greh?

Common Phrases for the Exam for Upper Gastrointestinal Bleeding

We are going to place a nasogastric tube.

Vamos a ponerle un tubo nasogástrico.
Bah-mohs ah poh-**nehr**-leh oon **too**-boh nah-soh-**gahs**-tree-koh.

Swallow when you feel the tube in your throat.

Trague cuando sienta el tubo en la garganta.
Trah-geh **kwahn**-doh see-**ehn**-tah ehl **too**-boh ehn lah gahr-**gahn**-tah.

You need a blood transfusion.

Usted necesita una transfusion de sangre.
Oos-**tehd** neh-seh-**see**-tah **oo**-nah trahns-foo-see-**ohn** deh **sahn**-greh.

You need intravenous fluids.

Usted necesita líquidos intravenosos.
Oos-**tehd** neh-seh-**see**-tah **lee**-kee-dohs een-trah-beh-**noh**-sohs.

We are going to admit you.

Lo / La vamos a internar.
Loh / Lah **bah**-mohs ah een-tehr-**nahr**.

Discharge Instructions for Upper Gastrointestinal Bleeding

Return to the hospital (clinic) if . . .

Regrese al hospital (a la clínica) si...
Reh-**greh**-seh ahl ohs-pee-**tahl** (ah lah **klee**-nee-kah) see...

you vomit blood,

vomita sangre,
boh-**mee**-tah **sahn**-greh,

you have abdominal pain,	tiene dolor abdominal, tee-**eh**-neh doh-**lohr** ab-doh-mee-**nahl**,
or you have black stools.	o tiene heces de color negro. oh tee-**eh**-neh **eh**-sehs deh koh-**lohr neh**-groh.
Avoid alcohol, aspirin, and spicy foods.	Evite las bebidas alcohólicas, la aspirina, y las comidas picantes. Eh-**bee**-teh lahs beh-**bee**-dahs ahl-**koh**-lee-kahs, lah ahs-pee-**ree**-nah, ee lahs koh-**mee**-dahs pee-**kahn**-tehs.
Take Maalox or Mylanta after each meal.	Tome Maalox o Mylanta después de cada comida. **Toh**-meh **Mah**-loks oh Mee-**lahn**-tah dehs-**pwehs** deh **kah**-dah koh-**mee**-dah.

Rectal Bleeding

Sangrado Rectal

Sahn-grah-doh rek-**tahl**

When did the bleeding start?	¿Cuándo empezó con el sangrado? **Kwahn**-doh ehm-peh-**soh** kohn ehl sahn-**grah**-doh?
Did you notice blood mixed with your stools?	¿Notó sangre mezclada con sus heces? Noh-**toh sahn**-greh mehs-**klah**-dah kohn soos **eh**-sehs?

Do you notice blood only when you wipe yourself?	¿Nota sangre solamente cuando se limpia? **Noh**-tah **sahn**-greh soh-lah-**mehn**-teh **kwahn**-doh seh **leem**-pee-ah?
Have you noticed blood in the toilet bowl?	¿Ha notado sangre en la taza del inodoro / retrete? Ah noh-**tah**-doh **sahn**-greh ehn lah **tah**-sah dehl ee-noh-**doh**-roh / reh-**treh**-teh?
What color is the blood?	¿De qué color es la sangre? Deh keh koh-**lohr** ehs lah **sahn**-greh?
Is it the color of fresh blood?	¿Es del color de sangre fresca? Ehs dehl koh-**lohr** deh **sahn**-greh **frehs**-kah?
Is it dark maroon?	¿Es un rojo obscuro? Ehs oon **roh**-ho ohbs-**koo**-roh?
Is it black?	¿Es negra? Ehs **neh**-grah?
What color are your stools?	¿De qué color son sus heces? Deh keh koh-**lohr** sohn soos **eh**-sehs?
Are they yellow?	¿Son amarillas? Sohn ah-mah-**ree**-yahs?
Are they dark brown?	¿Son de color café obscuro? Sohn de koh-**lohr** kah-**feh** ohbs-**koo**-roh?

Are they black?	¿Son negras? Sohn **neh**-grahs?
Do you drink alcohol?	¿Toma bebidas alcohólicas? **Toh**-mah beh-**bee**-dahs ahl-**koh**-lee-kahs?
Do you suffer from constipation?	¿Sufre usted de estreñimiento? **Soo**-freh oos-**tehd** deh ehs-treh-nyee-mee-**ehn**-toh?
Do you know if you have . . .	¿Sabe si tiene... **Sah**-beh see tee-**eh**-neh...
stomach ulcers?	úlceras del estómago? **ool**-seh-rahs dehl ehs-**toh**-mah-goh?
diverticulosis?	diverticulosis? dee-behr-tee-koo-**loh**-sees?
colon cancer?	cáncer del colon? **kahn**-sehr dehl **koh**-lohn?
hemorrhoids?	hemorroides? eh-moh-**roh**-ee-dehs?
Do you have abdominal pain?	¿Tiene usted dolor abdominal? Tee-**eh**-neh oos-**tehd** doh-**lohr** ab-doh-mee-**nahl**?
Do you have dizzy spells?	¿Tiene usted mareos? Tee-**eh**-neh oos-**tehd** mah-**reh**-ohs?
Do you have chest pain?	¿Tiene dolor del pecho? Tee-**ehn**-eh doh-**lohr** dehl **peh**-choh?
Do you have shortness of breath?	¿Tiene falta de aire? Tee-**ehn**-eh **fahl**-tah deh **ah**-ee-reh?

Do you have vomiting?	¿Tiene vómito? Tee-**eh**-neh **boh**-mee-toh?
Have you vomited blood?	¿Ha vomitado sangre? Ah boh-mee-**tah**-doh **sahn**-greh?
What color is the blood?	¿De qué color es la sangre? Deh keh koh-**lohr** ehs lah **sahn**-greh?
Is it the color of fresh blood?	¿Es del color de sangre fresca? Ehs dehl koh-**lohr** deh **sahn**-greh **frehs**-kah?
Is it brown?	¿Es de color café? Ehs deh koh-**lohr** kah-**feh**?
Is it black?	¿Es negra? Ehs **neh**-grah?

Common Phrases for the Exam for Rectal Bleeding

I need to do a rectal exam.	Necesito hacerle un examen del recto. Neh-seh-**see**-toh ah-**sehr**-leh oon ek-**sah**-mehn dehl **rek**-toh.
We are going to put in an intravenous line.	Vamos a ponerle una línea intravenosa. **Bah**-mohs ah poh-**nehr**-leh **oo**-nah **lee**-neh-ah een-trah-beh-**noh**-sah.

You need a blood transfusion.	Usted necesita una transfusión de sangre. Oos-**tehd** neh-seh-**see**-tah **oo**-nah trahns-foo-see-**ohn** deh **sahn**-greh.
You have hemorrhoids.	Usted tiene hemorrhoides. Oos-**tehd** tee-**eh**-neh eh-moh-**roh**-ee-dehs.
You have diverticulosis.	Usted tiene diverticulosis. Oos-**tehd** tee-**eh**-neh dee-behr-tee-koo-**loh**-sees.

Discharge Instructions for Rectal Bleeding

Return to the hospital (clinic) if . . .	Regrese al hospital (a la clínica) si tiene... Reh-**greh**-seh ahl ohs-pee-**tahl** (ah lah **klee**-nee-kah) see tee-**eh**-neh...
you have more bleeding,	más sangrado, mahs sahn-**grah**-doh,
you are dizzy,	mareos, mah-**reh**-ohs,
or you have chest pain.	o dolor del pecho. oh doh-**lohr** dehl **peh**-choh.

Urinary Retention

Retención Urinaria

Reh-tehn-see-**ohn** oo-ree-**nah**-ree-ah

When was the last time you urinated?

¿Cuándo fue la última vez que orinó?
Kwahn-doh fweh lah **ool**-tee-mah behs keh oh-ree-**noh**?

(X) hours (days) ago.

(X) horas (días).
(X) **oh**-rahs (**dee**-ahs).

Do you have abdominal pain?

¿Tiene dolor abdominal?
Tee-**eh**-neh doh-**lohr** ab-doh-mee-**nahl**?

Is your abdomen getting bigger?

¿Se está poniendo más grande su abdomen?
Seh ehs-**tah** poh-nee-**ehn**-doh mahs **grahn**-deh soo ab-**doh**-mehn?

Do you have a fever?

¿Tiene fiebre?
Tee-**eh**-neh fee-**eh**-breh?

Do you have nausea or vomiting?

¿Tiene náusea o vómito?
Tee-**eh**-neh **nah**-oo-seh-ah oh **boh**-mee-toh?

Do you have problems starting to urinate?

¿Tiene problemas al empezar a orinar?
Tee-**eh**-neh proh-**bleh**-mahs ahl ehm-peh-**sahr** ah oh-ree-**nahr**?

Do you dribble when you finish urinating?

¿Gotea al terminar de orinar?
Goh-**teh**-ah ahl tehr-mee-**nahr** deh oh-ree-**nahr**?

Does it burn when you urinate?	¿Tiene ardor al orinar? Tee-**eh**-neh ahr-**dohr** ahl oh-ree-**nahr**?
Have you noticed blood in your urine?	¿Ha notado sangre en la orina? Ah noh-**tah**-doh **sahn**-greh ehn lah oh-**ree**-nah?
(*For a man*) Have you had problems with your prostate?	¿Ha tenido problemas con su próstata? Ah teh-**nee**-doh proh-**bleh**-mahs kohn soo **prohs**-tah-tah?
Have you had venereal diseases?	¿Ha tenido enfermedades venéreas? Ah teh-**nee**-doh ehn-fehr-meh-**dah**-dehs beh-**neh**-reh-ahs?

Common Phrases for the Exam for Urinary Retention

You need a catheter in your bladder.	Usted necesita una sonda en la vejiga. Oos-**tehd** neh-seh-**see**-tah **oo**-nah **sohn**-dah ehn lah beh-**hee**-gah.
I need to examine your prostate.	Necesito examinar su próstata. Neh-seh-**see**-toh ek-sah-mee-**nahr** soo **prohs**-tah-tah.
Your prostate is very big.	Su próstata está muy grande. Soo **prohs**-tah-tah ehs-**tah** **moo**-ee **grahn**-deh.
You have a urinary tract infection.	Usted tiene una infección en la orina. Oos-**tehd** tee-**eh**-neh **oo**-nah een-fek-see-**ohn** ehn lah oh-**ree**-nah.

You have a prostate infection.

Usted tiene una infección de la próstata.
Oos-**tehd** tee-**eh**-neh **oo**-nah een-fek-see-**ohn** deh lah **prohs**-tah-tah.

You need to see a specialist.

Necesita ver a un especialista.
Neh-seh-**see**-tah behr ah oon ehs-peh-see-ah-**lees**-tah.

Discharge Instructions for Urinary Retention

Take your medication.

Tome su medicina.
Toh-meh soo meh-dee-**see**-nah.

Leave the catheter in your bladder until you see the specialist.

Deje la sonda en la vejiga hasta que vea al especialista.
Deh-heh lah **sohn**-dah ehn lah beh-**hee**-gah **ahs**-tah keh **beh**-ah ahl ehs-peh-see-ah-**lees**-tah.

Return to the hospital (clinic) if . . .

Regrese al hospital (a la clínica) si...
Reh-**greh**-seh ahl ohs-pee-**tahl** (ah lah **klee**-nee-kah) see...

you have fever or vomiting,

tiene fiebre o vómito,
tee-**eh**-neh fee-**eh**-breh oh **boh**-mee-toh,

you have abdominal pain,

tiene dolor abdominal,
tee-**eh**-neh doh-**lohr** ab-doh-mee-**nahl**,

or the catheter is blocked or falls out.

o la sonda está tapada o se sale.
oh lah **sohn**-dah ehs-**tah** tah-**pah**-dah oh seh **sah**-leh.

Hematuria

Sangre en la Orina

Sahn-greh ehn lah oh-**ree**-nah

When did you notice blood in your urine?

¿Cuándo notó sangre en la orina?
Kwahn-doh noh-**toh sahn**-greh ehn lah oh-**ree**-nah?

Have you had blood in your urine in the past?

¿Ha tenido sangre en la orina en el pasado?
Ah teh-**nee**-doh **sahn**-greh ehn lah oh-**ree**-nah ehn ehl pah-**sah**-doh?

Do you have pain in your abdomen?

¿Tiene dolor en el abdomen?
Tee-**eh**-neh doh-**lohr** ehn ehl ahb-**doh**-mehn?

Do you have pain in your testicles?

¿Tiene dolor en los testículos?
Tee-**eh**-neh doh-**lohr** ehn lohs tehs-**tee**-koo-lohs?

Do you have back pain?

¿Tiene dolor en la espalda?
Tee-**eh**-neh doh-**lohr** ehn lah ehs-**pahl**-dah?

Where did the pain start?

¿Dónde empezó el dolor?
Dohn-deh ehm-peh-**soh** ehl doh-**lohr**?

Does the pain travel to your abdomen (or testicles)?

¿Le viaja el dolor al abdomen (o a los testículos)?
Leh bee-**ah**-hah ehl doh-**lohr** ahl abh-**doh**-mehn (oh ah lohs tehs-**tee**-koo-lohs)?

Do you have a fever?

¿Tiene fiebre?
Tee-**eh**-neh fee-**eh**-breh?

Do you have chills?	¿Tiene escalofríos? Tee-**eh**-neh ehs-kah-loh-**free**-ohs?
Do you have vomiting?	¿Tiene vómito? Tee-**eh**-neh **boh**-mee-toh?
How many times have you vomited?	¿Cuántas veces ha vomitado? **Kwahn**-tahs **beh**-sehs ah boh-mee-**tah**-doh?
Do you have difficulty urinating?	¿Tiene dificultades para orinar? Tee-**eh**-neh dee-fee-kool-**tah**-dehs **pah**-rah oh-ree-**nahr**?
Does it burn when you urinate?	¿Le arde cuando orina? Leh **ahr**-deh **kwahn**-doh oh-**ree**-nah?
Do you urinate more than normal?	¿Orina más de lo normal? Oh-**ree**-nah mahs deh loh nohr-**mahl**?
Do you have a discharge from your penis?	¿Tiene deshecho del pene? Tee-**eh**-neh dehs-**eh**-choh dehl **peh**-neh?
Do you have a discharge from your vagina?	¿Tiene deshecho de la vagina? Tee-**eh**-neh dehs-**eh**-choh deh lah bah-**hee**-nah?
Have you had bladder or kidney infections?	¿Ha tenido infecciones de la vejiga o de los riñones? Ah teh-**nee**-doh een-fek-see-**oh**-nehs deh lah beh-**hee**-gah oh deh los ree-**nyoh**-nehs?
Do you suffer from kidney stones?	¿Sufre usted de cálculos en los riñones? **Soo**-freh oos-**tehd** deh **kahl**-koo-lohs ehn lohs ree-**nyoh**-nehs?

Have you lost weight?

¿Ha perdido peso?
Ah pehr-**dee**-doh **peh**-soh?

Common Phrases for the Exam for Hematuria

We need a urine sample.

Necesitamos una muestra de orina.
Neh-seh-see-**tah**-mohs **oo**-nah **mwehs**-trah deh oh-**ree**-nah.

We need an ultrasound of your kidneys.

Necesitamos hacerle un ultrasonido de los riñones.
Neh-seh-see-**tah**-mos ah-**sehr**-leh oon ool-trah-soh-**nee**-doh deh lohs ree-**nyoh**-nehs.

You need an IVP (a photograph of your kidneys).

Usted necesita un IVP (una fotografía de los riñones).
Oos-**tehd** neh-seh-**see**-tah oon eye vee pee (**oo**-nah foh-toh-**grah**-fee-ah deh lohs ree-**nyoh**-nehs).

Are you allergic to shrimp or iodine?

Es alérgico / -a a los camarones o al iodo?
Ehs ah-**lehr**-hee-koh / -kah ah lohs kah-mah-**roh**-nehs oh ahl **yoh**-doh?

We need to put a catheter in your bladder.

Necesitamos ponerle una sonda en la vejiga.
Neh-seh-see-**tah**-mohs poh-**nehr**-leh **oo**-nah **sohn**-dah ehn lah beh-**hee**-gah.

I am going to give you pain medicine.

Le voy a dar medicina para el dolor.
Leh **boh**-ee ah dahr meh-dee-**see**-nah **pah**-rah ehl doh-**lohr**.

You have a kidney stone.

Usted tiene una piedra (un cálculo) en el riñón.
Oos-**tehd** tee-**eh**-neh **oo**-nah pee-**eh**-drah (oon **kahl**-koo-loh) ehn ehl ree-**nyohn**.

You have an obstruction in your kidney caused by a calculus.

Usted tiene una obstrucción en el riñón causada por una piedra (un cálculo).
Oos-**tehd** tee-**eh**-neh **oo**-nah obs-truk-see-**ohn** ehn ehl ree-**nyohn** kah-oo-**sah**-dah pohr **oo**-nah pee-**eh**-drah (oon **kahl**-koo-loh).

You passed a kidney stone.

Usted pasó una piedra (un cálculo) renal.
Oos-**tehd** pah-**soh** oo-nah pee-**eh**-drah (oon **kahl**-koo-loh) reh-**nahl**.

Discharge Instructions for Hematuria

Drink a lot of fluids.

Tome muchos líquidos.
Toh-meh **moo**-chohs **lee**-kee-dohs.

Return to the hospital (clinic) if you have . . .

Regrese al hospital (a la clínica) si tiene...
Reh-**greh**-seh ahl ohs-pee-**tahl** (ah lah **klee**-nee-kah) see tee-**eh**-neh...

constant pain,

dolor constante,
doh-**lohr** kohns-**tahn**-teh,

persistent vomiting,

vómito persistente,
boh-mee-toh pehr-sis-**tehn**-teh,

difficulty urinating,

dificultades para orinar,
dee-fee-kool-**tah**-dehs
pah-rah oh-ree-**nahr**,

or fever.

o fiebre.
oh fee-**eh**-breh.

You have to strain your urine and see if there are stones.

Es necesario que cuele la orina para ver si hay piedras.
Ehs neh-seh-**sah**-ree-oh keh **kweh**-leh lah oh-**ree**-nah **pah**-rah behr see **ah**-ee pee-**eh**-drahs.

Scrotal Pain

Dolor en el Escroto

Doh-**lohr** ehn ehl ehs-**kroh**-toh

When did the pain start?

¿Cuándo empezó el dolor?
Kwahn-doh ehm-peh-**soh** ehl doh-**lohr**?

In which testicle do you have the pain?

¿En cuál testículo tiene el dolor?
Ehn kwahl tehs-**tee**-koo-loh tee-**eh**-neh ehl doh-**lohr**?

Have you had a similar pain in the past?

¿Ha tenido dolor similar en el pasado?
Ah teh-**nee**-doh doh-**lohr** see-mee-**lahr** ehn ehl pah-**sah**-doh?

When?

¿Cuándo?
Kwahn-doh?

Do you have swelling in the testicle?

¿Tiene hinchazón en el testículo?
Tee-**eh**-neh een-chah-**sohn** ehn ehl tehs-**tee**-koo-loh?

Did you receive a blow to the testicle?	¿Recibió un golpe al testículo? Reh-see-bee-**oh** oon **gohl**-peh ahl tehs-**tee**-koo-loh?
Did you lift anything heavy?	¿Levantó algo pesado? Leh-bahn-**toh ahl**-goh peh-**sah**-doh?
Do you have a discharge from the penis?	¿Tiene deshecho del pene? Tee-**eh**-neh dehs-**eh**-choh dehl **peh**-neh?
Does it burn when you urinate?	¿Tiene ardor al orinar? Tee-**eh**-neh ahr-**dohr** ahl oh-ree-**nahr**?
Do you have a fever?	¿Tiene fiebre? Tee-**eh**-neh fee-**eh**-breh?
Do you have abdominal pain?	¿Tiene dolor abdominal? Tee-**eh**-neh doh-**lohr** abh-doh-mee-**nahl**?
Do you have nausea or vomiting?	¿Tiene náusea o vómito? Tee-**eh**-neh **nah**-oo-seh-ah oh **boh**-mee-toh?
With how many people do you have sex?	¿Con cuántas personas tiene sexo? Kohn **kwahn**-tahs pehr-**soh**-nahs tee-**eh**-neh **sek**-soh?
Do you use condoms . . .	¿Usa condones / preservativos... **Oo**-sah kohn-**doh**-nehs / preh-sehr-bah-**tee**-bohs...
always?	siempre? see-**ehm**-preh?
sometimes?	a veces? ah **beh**-sehs?

never?	nunca? **noon**-kah?
Have you had venereal diseases in the past?	¿Ha tenido enfermedades venéreas en el pasado? Ah teh-**nee**-doh ehn-fehr-meh-**dah**-dehs beh-**neh**-reh-ahs ehn ehl pah-**sah**-doh?
Have you had . . .	¿Ha tenido... Ah teh-**nee**-doh...
gonorrhea?	gonorrea? goh-noh-**reh**-ah?
syphilis?	sífilis? **see**-fee-lees?
trichomonas?	tricomonas? Tree-koh-**moh**-nahs?
chlamydia?	clamidia? Klah-**mee**-dee-ah?
herpes?	herpes? **ehr**-pehs?

Common Phrases for the Exam for Scrotal Pain

I need to examine your penis and testicles.	Necesito examinarle el pene y los testículos. Neh-seh-**see**-toh ek-sah-mee-**nahr** ehl **peh**-neh ee lohs tehs-**tee**-koo-lohs.
I need to do penile cultures.	Necesito hacerle cultivos del pene. Neh-seh-**see**-toh ah-**sehr**-leh kool-**tee**-bohs dehl **peh**-neh.

I need a urine sample.

Necesito una muestra de orina.
Neh-seh-**see**-toh **oo**-nah **mwehs**-trah deh oh-**ree**-nah.

You need intravenous antibiotics.

Usted necesita antibióticos intravenosos.
Oos-**tehd** neh-seh-**see**-tah ahn-tee-bee-**oh**-tee-kohs een-trah-beh-**noh**-sohs.

You need an injection.

Usted necesita una inyección.
Oos-**tehd** neh-seh-**see**-tah **oo**-nah een-yek-see-**ohn**.

You have an infection in your testicles.

Tiene una infección en los testículos.
Tee-**eh**-neh **oo**-nah een-fek-see-**ohn** ehn lohs tehs-**tee**-koo-lohs.

Discharge Instructions for Scrotal Pain

Take one pill of your medicine every (X) hours.

Tome una pastilla de su medicina cada (X) horas.
Toh-meh **oo**-nah pahs-**tee**-yah deh soo meh-dee-**see**-nah **kah**-dah (X) **oh**-rahs.

Return to the hospital (clinic) if you have . . .

Regrese al hospital (a la clínica) si tiene...
Reh-**greh**-seh ahl ohs-pee-**tahl** (ah lah **klee**-nee-kah) see tee-**eh**-neh...

a fever,

fiebre,
fee-**eh**-breh,

abdominal pain or vomiting,

dolor abdominal o vómito,
doh-**lohr** abh-doh-mee-**nahl** oh **boh**-mee-toh,

or more scrotal pain.

o más dolor en el escroto.
oh mahs doh-**lohr** ehn ehl ehs-**kroh**-toh.

Don't have sex without condoms.

No tenga sexo sin condones / preservativos.
Noh **tehn**-gah **sek**-soh seen kohn-**doh**-nehs / preh-sehr-bah-**tee**-bohs.

Penile Discharge

Deshecho del Pene

Dehs-**eh**-choh dehl **peh**-neh

How many days have you had the discharge?

¿Por cuántos días ha tenido el deshecho?
Pohr **kwahn**-tohs **dee**-ahs ah teh-**nee**-doh ehl dehs-**eh**-choh?

Do you have burning when you urinate?

¿Tiene ardor al orinar?
Tee-**eh**-neh ahr-**dohr** ahl oh-ree-**nahr**?

Have you noticed blood in your urine?

¿Ha notado sangre en la orina?
Ah noh-**tah**-doh **sahn**-greh ehn lah oh-**ree**-nah?

Do you have pain in your testicles?

¿Tiene dolor en los testículos?
Tee-**eh**-neh doh-**lohr** ehn lohs tehs-**tee**-koo-lohs?

Do you have abdominal pain?

¿Tiene dolor abdominal?
Tee-**eh**-neh doh-**lohr** abh-doh-mee-**nahl**?

Do you have a fever?

¿Tiene fiebre?
Tee-**eh**-neh fee-**eh**-breh?

Have you had venereal diseases in the past?	¿Ha tenido enfermedades venéreas en el pasado? Ah teh-**nee**-doh ehn-fehr-meh-**dah**-dehs beh-**neh**-reh-ahs ehn ehl pah-**sah**-doh?
Have you had . . .	¿Ha tenido... Ah teh-**nee**-doh...
gonorrhea?	gonorrea? goh-noh-**reh**-ah?
syphilis?	sífilis? **see**-fee-lees?
trichomonas?	tricomonas? Tree-koh-**moh**-nahs?
chlamydia?	clamidia? Klah-**mee**-dee-ah?
herpes?	herpes? **ehr**-pehs?
With how many people do you have sex?	¿Con cuántas personas tiene sexo? Kohn **kwahn**-tahs pehr-**soh**-nahs tee-**eh**-neh **sek**-soh?
Do you have sexual relations with men (women, prostitutes)?	¿Tiene usted relaciones sexuales con hombres (mujeres, prostitutas)? Tee-**eh**-neh oos-**tehd** reh-lah-see-**oh**-nehs sek-soo-**ah**-lehs kohn **ohm**-brehs (moo-**heh**-rehs, prohs-tee-**too**-tahs)?
Do you use condoms?	¿Usa condones / preservativos? **Oo**-sah kohn-**doh**-nehs / preh-sehr-bah-**tee**-bohs?

Have you had an AIDS test?	¿Ha tenido una prueba del SIDA?
	Ah teh-**nee**-doh **oo**-nah **prweh**-bah dehl **see**-dah?
What are the HIV results?	¿Cuales son los resultados del HIV?
	Kwah-lehs sohn lohs reh-sool-**tah**-dohs dehl ache-ee-beh?
Positive?	¿Positivos?
	Poh-see-**tee**-bohs?
Negative?	¿Negativos?
	Neh-gah-**tee**-bohs?
You don't know?	¿No sabe?
	Noh **sah**-beh?

Common Phrases for the Exam for Penile Discharge

I need to examine your penis and testicles.	Necesito examinarle el pene y los testículos.
	Neh-seh-**see**-toh ek-sah-mee-**nahr**-leh ehl **peh**-neh ee lohs tehs-**tee**-koo-lohs.
I need to take some penile cultures.	Necesito hacerle cultivos del pene.
	Neh-seh-**see**-toh ah-**sehr**-leh kool-**tee**-bohs dehl **peh**-neh.
I need a urine sample.	Necesito una muestra de orina.
	Neh-seh-**see**-toh **oo**-nah **mwehs**-trah deh oh-**ree**-nah.

You have a venereal disease.

Usted tiene una enfermedad
venérea.
Oos-**tehd** tee-**eh**-neh **oo**-nah
ehn-fehr-meh-**dahd** beh-**neh**-
reh-ah.

I am going to give you an
antibiotic injection.

Le voy a dar una inyección de
antibiótico.
Leh **boh**-ee ah dahr **oo**-nah
een-yek-see-**ohn** deh ahn-tee-
bee-**oh**-tee-koh.

Discharge Instructions for Penile Discharge

Inform all of your sexual
partners about your condition.

Informe a todas sus parejas
sexuales acerca de su
condición.
Een-**fohr**-meh ah **toh**-dahs
soos pah-**reh**-has sehk-soo-**ah**-
les ah-**sehr**-kah deh soo kohn-
dee-see-**ohn**.

Use condoms whenever you
have sex.

Use condones / preservativos
cada vez que tenga relaciones
sexuales.
Oo-seh kohn-**doh**-nehs / preh-
sehr-bah-**tee**-bohs **kah**-dah
behs keh **tehn**-gah reh-lah-see-
oh-nes sehk-soo-**ah**-les.

Take (X) pills of your
medicine every (Y) hours.

Tome (X) pastillas de su
medicina cada (Y) horas.
Toh-meh (X) pahs-**tee**-yahs
deh soo meh-dee-**see**-nah **kah**-
dah (Y) **oh**-rahs.

The Dialysis Patient

El Paciente de Diálisis

Ehl pah-see-**ehn**-teh deh dee-**ah**-lee-sees

Are you short of breath?

¿Tiene falta de aire?
Tee-**eh**-neh **fahl**-tah deh **ah**-ee-reh?

When did the shortness of breath start?

¿Cuándo empezó la falta de aire?
Kwahn-doh ehm-peh-**soh** lah **fahl**-tah deh **ah**-ee-reh?

(X) hours (days) ago.

(X) horas (días).
(X) **oh**-rahs (**dee**-ahs).

Do you have chest pain?

¿Tiene dolor en el pecho?
Tee-**eh**-neh doh-**lohr** ehn ehl **peh**-choh?

Do you feel weak?

¿Se siente débil?
Seh see-**ehn**-teh **deh**-beel?

When was the last time you had dialysis?

¿Cuándo fue la última vez que tuvo diálisis?
Kwahn-doh fweh lah **ool**-tee-mah behs keh **too**-boh dee-**ah**-lee-sees?

How many times a week do you have dialysis?

¿Cuántas veces a la semana tiene diálisis?
Kwahn-tahs **beh**-sehs ah lah seh-**mah**-nah tee-**eh**-neh dee-**ah**-lee-sees?

Have you missed a day of
dialysis this week?

¿Ha faltado algún día de
diálisis esta semana?
Ah fahl-**tah**-doh ahl-**goon dee**-
ah deh dee-**ah**-lee-sees **ehs**-tah
seh-**mah**-nah?

How many months (years)
have you been on dialysis?

¿Cuántos meses (años) tiene
con diálisis?
Kwahn-tohs **meh**-sehs (**ah**-
nyohs) tee-**eh**-neh kohn dee-
ah-lee-sees?

Are you producing urine?

¿Puede hacer orina?
Pweh-deh ah-**sehr** oh-**ree**-nah?

Are you making a small
(normal) amount?

¿Hace una cantidad
pequeña (normal)?
Ah-seh **oo**-nah kahn-tee-
dahd peh-**keh**-nyah (nohr-
mahl)?

When was the last time you
urinated?

¿Cuándo fue la última vez que
orinó?
Kwahn-doh fweh lah **ool**-tee-
mah behs keh oh-ree-**noh**?

Have they intubated you for
excess fluid in your body?

¿Lo / La han intubado por
exceso de agua en su cuerpo?
Loh / Lah ahn een-too-**bah**-doh
pohr ek-**seh**-soh deh **ah**-gwah
ehn soo **kwehr**-poh?

Do you have a fever?

¿Tiene fiebre?
Tee-**eh**-neh fee-**eh**-breh?

Do you have nausea or
vomiting?

¿Tiene náusea o vómito?
Tee-**eh**-neh **nah**-oo-seh-ah oh
boh-mee-toh?

Do you have diabetes?

¿Tiene diabetes?
Tee-**eh**-neh dee-ah-**beh**-tehs?

Do you have high blood pressure?	¿Tiene alta presión de la sangre? Tee-**eh**-neh **ahl**-tah preh-see-**ohn** deh lah **sahn**-greh?
What medicine do you take?	¿Qué medicina toma? Keh meh-dee-**see**-nah **toh**-mah?
Do you follow a special diet?	¿Sigue una dieta especial? **See**-geh **oo**-nah dee-**eh**-tah ehs-peh-see-**ahl**?

Common Phrases for the Exam of the Dialysis Patient

You need dialysis today.	Usted necesita diálisis hoy. Oos-**tehd** neh-seh-**see**-tah dee-**ah**-lee-sees **oh**-ee.
You need to be intubated.	Usted necesita intubación. Oos-**tehd** neh-seh-**see**-tah een-too-bah-see-**ohn**.
We are going to admit you to do dialysis.	Vamos a internarlo / -la para hacerle diálisis. **Bah**-mohs ah een-tehr-**nahr**-loh / -lah **pah**-rah ah-**sehr**-leh dee-**ah**-lee-sees.
You don't need dialysis yet.	Todavía no necesita diálisis. Toh-dah-**bee**-ah noh neh-seh-**see**-tah dee-**ah**-lee-sees.

Discharge Instructions for the Dialysis Patient

Return to the hospital (clinic) if . . .	Regrese al hospital (a la clínica) si... Reh-**greh**-seh ahl ohs-pee-**tahl** (ah lah **klee**-nee-kah) see...

you have shortness of breath,

tiene falta de aire,
tee-**eh**-neh **fahl**-tah deh **ah**-ee-reh,

you have chest pain,

tiene dolor del pecho,
tee-**eh**-neh doh-**lohr** dehl **peh**-choh,

or your body swells up.

o se le hincha el cuerpo.
oh seh leh **een**-chah ehl **kwehr**-poh.

Don't miss your dialysis appointment.

No falte a su cita de diálisis.
Noh **fahl**-teh ah soo **see**-tah deh dee-**ah**-lee-sees.

Obstetrics/Gynecology

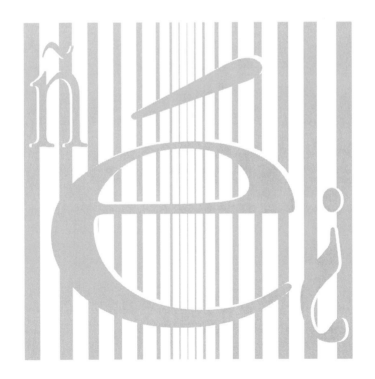

Vaginal Discharge

Deshecho Vaginal

Dehs-eh-choh bah-hee-nahl

How long have you had the discharge?	¿Cuánto tiempo tiene con el deshecho / flujo? **Kwahn-toh tee-ehm-poh tee-eh-neh kohn ehl dehs-eh-choh / floo-hoh?**
What color is the discharge?	¿De qué color es el deshecho? **Deh keh koh-lohr ehs ehl dehs-eh-choh?**
Is it white?	¿Es blanco? **Ehs blahn-koh?**
Is it yellow?	¿Es amarillo? **Ehs ah-mah-ree-yoh?**
Is it brown?	¿Es de color café? **Ehs deh koh-lohr kah-feh?**
Do you have itching?	¿Tiene comezón? **Tee-eh-neh koh-meh-sohn?**
Does the discharge have a bad odor?	¿Tiene mal olor el deshecho? **Tee-eh-neh mahl oh-lohr ehl dehs-eh-choh?**
Do you have abdominal pain?	¿Tiene dolor abdominal? **Tee-eh-neh doh-lohr abh-doh-mee-nahl?**
Do you have a fever?	¿Tiene fiebre? **Tee-eh-neh fee-eh-breh?**
Do you have burning when you urinate?	¿Tiene ardor al orinar? **Tee-eh-neh ahr-dohr ahl oh-ree-nahr?**

| With how many people do you have sex? | ¿Con cuántas personas tiene sexo? |
| | Kohn **kwahn**-tahs pehr-**soh**-nahs tee-**eh**-neh **sek**-soh? |

| Do you have a new boyfriend? | ¿Tiene un novio nuevo? |
| | Tee-**eh**-neh oon **noh**-bee-oh **nweh**-boh? |

| When was your last period? | ¿Cuándo fue su última regla / menstruación? |
| | **Kwahn**-doh fweh soo **ool**-tee-mah **reh**-glah / mehns-troo-ah-see-**ohn**? |

| Month? | ¿El mes? |
| | Ehl mehs? |

| Day? | ¿El día? |
| | Ehl **dee**-ah? |

| Year? | ¿El año? |
| | Ehl **ah**-nyoh? |

| How many times have you been pregnant? | ¿Cuántas veces ha estado embarazada? |
| | **Kwahn**-tahs **beh**-sehs ah ehs-**tah**-doh ehm-bah-rah-**sah**-dah? |

| How many children do you have? | ¿Cuántos hijos tiene? |
| | **Kwahn**-tohs **ee**-hohs tee-**eh**-neh? |

| Have you had vaginal infections? | ¿Ha tenido infecciones vaginales? |
| | Ah teh-**nee**-doh een-fek-see-**oh**-nehs bah-hee-**nah**-lehs? |

| Have you had venereal diseases in the past? | ¿Ha tenido enfermedades venéreas en el pasado? |
| | Ah teh-**nee**-doh ehn-fehr-meh-**dah**-dehs beh-**neh**-reh-ahs ehn ehl pah-**sah**-doh? |

Have you had . . . | ¿Ha tenido...
| Ah teh-**nee**-doh...

gonorrhea? | gonorrea?
| goh-noh-**reh**-ah?

syphilis? | sífilis?
| **see**-fee-lees?

trichomonas? | tricomonas?
| Tree-koh-**moh**-nahs?

chlamydia? | clamidia?
| Klah-**mee**-dee-ah?

herpes? | herpes?
| **ehr**-pehs?

Do you always use condoms? | ¿Siempre usa condones /
| preservativos?
| See-**ehm**-preh **oo**-sah kohn-
| **doh**-nehs / preh-sehr-bah-**tee**-
| bohs?

Are you allergic to penicillin,
tetracycline, or sulfa? | ¿Es alérgica a la penicilina,
| tetraciclina, o sulfa?
| Ehs ah-**lehr**-hee-kah ah lah
| peh-nee-see-**lee**-nah, teh-trah-
| see-**klee**-nah, oh **sool**-fah?

Common Phrases for the Exam for Vaginal Discharge

I need to do a vaginal exam. | Necesito hacerle un examen
| vaginal.
| Neh-seh-**see**-toh ah-**sehr**-leh
| oon ek-**sah**-mehn bah-hee-
| **nahl**.

I need to take some vaginal cultures.	Necesito hacerle unos cultivos vaginales. Neh-seh-**see**-toh ah-**sehr**-leh **oo**-nohs kool-**tee**-bohs bah-hee-**nah**-lehs.
You have . . .	Usted tiene... Oos-**tehd** tee-**eh**-neh...
yeast / candida.	hongos / candida. **ohn**-gohs / kahn-**dee**-dah.
chlamydia.	clamidia. Klah-**mee**-dee-ah.
gardnerella.	gardnerella. gahrd-neh-**reh**-lah.
trichomonas.	tricomonas. Tree-koh-**moh**-nahs.
pelvic inflammatory disease.	enfermedad inflamatoria de la pelvis. ehn-fehr-meh-**dahd** een-flah-mah-**toh**-ree-ah deh lah **pehl**-bees.
I need to give you an injection.	Es necesario ponerle una inyección. Ehs neh-seh-**sah**-ree-oh poh-**nehr**-leh **oo**-nah een-yek-see-**ohn**.
You need intravenous antibiotics.	Usted necesita antibióticos intravenosos. Oos-**tehd** neh-seh-**see**-tah ahn-tee-bee-**oh**-tee-kohs een-trah-beh-**noh**-sohs.
We are going to admit you.	Vamos a internarla. **Bah**-mohs ah een-tehr-**nahr**-lah.

Discharge Instructions for Vaginal Discharge

Use the cream every night
before going to bed.

Use la crema todas las noches
antes de acostarse.
Oo-seh lah **kreh**-mah **toh**-dahs
lahs **noh**-chehs **ahn**-tehs deh
ah-kohs-**tahr**-seh.

Take one pill every twelve
hours.

Tome una pastilla cada doce
horas.
Toh-meh **oo**-nah pahs-**tee**-yah
kah-dah **doh**-seh **oh**-rahs.

You must inform your
partners of your condition.

Debe informarles a sus parejas
de su condición.
Deh-beh een-fohr-**mahr**-lehs ah
soos pah-**reh**-hahs deh soo
kohn-dee-see-**ohn**.

Your partners must also
receive medical treatment.

Sus parejas también deben
recibir tratamiento médico.
Soos pah-**reh**-hahs tahm-bee-
ehn deh-behn reh-see-**beer**
trah-tah-mee-**ehn**-toh **meh**-dee-
koh.

Don't have sex for two weeks.

No tenga sexo por dos
semanas.
Noh **tehn**-gah **sek**-soh pohr
dohs seh-**mah**-nahs.

Use condoms.

Use condones / preservativos.
Oo-seh kohn-**doh**-nehs / preh-
sehr-bah-**tee**-bohs.

Vaginal Bleeding

Sangrado Vaginal

Sahn-grah-doh bah-**hee**-nahl

When was your last period / menstruation?

¿Cuándo fue su última regla / menstruación?
Kwahn-doh fweh soo **ool**-tee-mah **reh**-glah / mehns-troo-ah-see-**ohn**?

Month?

¿El mes?
Ehl mehs?

Day?

¿El día?
Ehl **dee**-ah?

Year?

¿El año?
Ehl **ah**-nyoh?

Are you pregnant?

¿Esta embarazada?
Ehs-**tah** ehm-bah-rah-**sah**-dah?

How many months along are you?

¿Cuántos meses tiene?
Kwahn-tohs **meh**-sehs tee-**eh**-neh?

How many times have you been pregnant?

¿Cuántas veces ha estado embarazada?
Kwahn-tahs **beh**-sehs ah ehs-**tah**-doh ehm-bah-rah-**sah**-dah?

How many times have you delivered?

¿Cuántas veces ha dado a luz?
Kwahn-tahs **beh**-sehs ah **dah**-doh ah loos?

How many premature babies have you had?

¿Cuántos bebés prematuros ha tenido?
Kwahn-tohs beh-**behs** preh-mah-**too**-rohs ah teh-**nee**-doh?

How many miscarriages (spontaneous abortions) have you had?

¿Cuántos malpartos (abortos espontáneos) ha tenido?
Kwahn-tohs mahl-**pahr**-tohs (ah-**bohr**-tohs ehs-pohn-**tah**-neh-ohs) ah teh-**nee**-doh?

How many induced abortions have you had?

¿Cuántos abortos provocados ha tenido?
Kwahn-tohs ah-**bohr**-tohs proh-boh-**kah**-dohs ah teh-**nee**-doh?

How many living children do you have?

¿Cuántos niños vivos tiene?
Kwahn-tohs **nee**-nyohs **bee**-bohs tee-**eh**-neh?

How long have you had vaginal bleeding?

¿Por cuánto tiempo ha tenido sangrado vaginal?
Pohr **kwahn**-toh tee-**ehm**-poh ah teh-**nee**-doh sahn-**grah**-doh bah-hee-**nahl**?

For (X) days (weeks, months).

Desde (X) días (semanas, meses).
Dehs-deh (X) **dee**-ahs (seh-**mah**-nahs, **meh**-sehs).

Did it happen after a fall?

¿Ocurrió después de caerse?
Oh-koo-ree-**oh** des-**pwehs** deh kah-**ehr**-seh?

Did it happen after having sex?

¿Ocurrió después de tener relaciones sexuales?
Oh-koo-ree-**oh** dehs-**pwehs** deh teh-**nehr** reh-lah-see-**oh**-nehs sek-soo-**ah**-lehs?

Did it happen after douching?	¿Ocurrió después de usar una ducha vaginal?
	Oh-koo-ree-**oh** des-**pwehs** deh oo-**sahr oo**-nah **doo**-chah bah-hee-**nahl**?
Is the vaginal bleeding constant?	¿Es el sangrado vaginal constante?
	Ehs ehl sahn-**grah**-doh bah-hee-**nahl** kohns-**tahn**-teh?
Is the vaginal bleeding intermittent?	¿El sangrado vaginal va y viene?
	Ehl sahn-**grah**-doh bah-hee-**nahl** bah ee bee-**eh**-neh?
Have you passed blood clots?	¿Ha arrojado coágulos de sangre?
	Ah ah-roh-**ha**-doh koh-**ah**-goo-lohs deh **sahn**-greh?
Have you passed tissue?	¿Ha pasado carnosidad / tejido?
	Ah pah-**sah**-doh kahr-noh-see-**dad** / teh-**hee**-doh?
How many sanitary pads did you use today?	¿Cuántas toallas femininas usó hoy?
	Kwahn-tahs toh-**ah**-yahs feh-meh-**nee**-nahs oo-**soh oh**-ee?
Do you have pain in your belly or stomach?	¿Tiene dolor en el vientre o estómago?
	Tee-**eh**-neh doh-**lohr** ehn ehl bee-**ehn**-treh oh ehs-**toh**-mah-goh?
Is the pain constant?	¿Es el dolor constante?
	Ehs ehl doh-**lohr** kohns-**tahn**-teh?

Does the pain come and go?	¿El dolor le va y viene? Ehl doh-**lohr** leh bah ee bee-**eh**-neh?
How long does the pain last?	¿Cuánto tiempo le dura el dolor? **Kwahn**-toh tee-**ehm**-poh leh **doo**-rah ehl doh-**lohr**?
Does the pain stay in one place?	¿El dolor se queda en un solo lugar? Ehl doh-**lohr** seh **keh**-dah ehn oon **soh**-loh loo-**gahr**?
Does the pain travel to another place?	¿El dolor le viaja a otro lado? Ehl doh-**lohr** leh bee-**ah**-ha ah **oh**-troh **lah**-doh?
Do you have cramps in your belly?	¿Tiene calambres / retortijones en el vientre? Tee-**eh**-neh kah-**lahm**-brehs / reh-tohr-tee-**ho**-nehs ehn ehl bee-**ehn**-treh?
Do you have nausea or vomiting?	¿Tiene náusea o vómito? Tee-**eh**-neh **nah**-oo-seh-ah oh **boh**-mee-toh?
Do you have diarrhea?	¿Tiene diarrea? Tee-**eh**-neh dee-ah-**reh**-ah?
Do you have a fever?	¿Tiene fiebre? Tee-**eh**-neh fee-**eh**-breh?
Do you feel dizzy?	¿Se siente mareada? Seh see-**ehn**-teh mah-reh-**ah**-dah?
Do you have back pain?	¿Tiene dolor en la espalda? Tee-**eh**-neh doh-**lohr** ehn lah ehs-**pahl**-dah?

Do you have a vaginal discharge?	¿Tiene flujo vaginal? Tee-**eh**-neh **floo**-hoh bah-hee-**nahl**?
What color is it?	¿De qué color es? Deh keh koh-**lohr** ehs?
Is it yellow?	¿Es amarilla? Ehs ah-mah-**ree**-yah?
Is it white?	¿Es blanca? Ehs **blahn**-kah?
Is it brown?	¿Es de color café? Ehs deh koh-**lohr** kah-**feh**?
Are you urinating more than normal?	¿Orina más de lo normal? Oh-**ree**-nah mahs deh loh nohr-**mahl**?
Do you have burning when you urinate?	¿Tiene ardor al orinar? Tee-**eh**-neh ahr-**dohr** ahl oh-ree-**nahr**?
Do you have pain when you urinate?	¿Tiene dolor al orinar? Tee-**eh**-neh doh-**lohr** ahl oh-ree-**nahr**?
Are you allergic to any medicine or food?	¿Es alérgica a alguna medicina o alimento? Ehs ah-**lehr**-hee-kah ah ahl-**goo**-nah meh-dee-**see**-nah oh ah-lee-**mehn**-toh?
What medicine have you taken for the pain?	¿Qué medicina ha tomado para el dolor? Keh meh-dee-**see**-nah ah toh-**mah**-doh **pah**-rah ehl doh-**lohr**?
Do you have . . .	¿Tiene usted de... Tee-**eh**-neh oos-**tehd** deh...

anemia?	anemia? ah-**neh**-mee-ah?
epileptic attacks?	ataques epilépticos? ah-**tah**-kehs eh-pee-**lep**-tee-kohs?
hypertension?	alta presión de la sangre? **ahl**-tah preh-see-**ohn** deh lah **sahn**-greh?
cancer?	cáncer? **kahn**-sehr?
diabetes?	diabetes? dee-ah-**beh**-tehs?
heart disease?	alguna enfermedad del corazón? ahl-**goo**-nah ehn-fehr-meh-**dad** dehl koh-rah-**sohn**?
kidney disease?	alguna enfermedad del riñón? ahl-**goo**-nah ehn-fehr-meh-**dad** dehl ree-**nyohn**?
Have you had . . .	¿Alguna vez le han... ¿Ahl-**goo**-nah behs leh ahn...
breast surgery?	operado de los senos? oh-peh-**rah**-doh deh lohs **seh**-nohs?
uterine surgery?	operado de la matriz / el útero? oh-peh-**rah**-doh deh lah **mah**-trees / ehl **oo**-teh-roh?

a D & C?	hecho un raspado / legrado del útero? **eh**-choh oon rahs-**pah**-doh / leh-**grah**-doh dehl **oo**-teh-roh?
At what age did you start having your periods?	¿A qué edad comenzó a reglar / menstruar? Ah keh eh-**dahd** koh-mehn-**soh** ah reh-**glahr** / mehns-troo-**ahr**?
Are your periods regular?	¿Sus reglas / menstruaciones son regulares? Soos **reh**-glahs / mehns-troo-ah-see-**oh**-nehs sohn reh-goo-**lah**-rehs?
How often do you menstruate, every month?	¿Qué tan seguido le viene la menstruación, cada mes? Keh tahn seh-**gee**-doh leh bee-**eh**-nehn lah mehns-troo-ah-see-**ohn**, **kah**-dah mehs?
Have you ever had . . .	Alguna vez ha tenido... Ahl-**goo**-nah behs ah teh-**nee**-doh...
gonorrhea?	gonorrea? goh-noh-**reh**-ah?
a tubal infection?	infección en un tubo? een-fek-see-**ohn** ehn oon **too**-boh?
syphilis?	sífilis? **see**-fee-lees?
a pelvic infection?	una infección pélvica? **oo**-nah een-fek-see-**ohn** **pehl**-bee-kah?
herpes?	herpes? **ehr**-pehs?

chlamydia?	clamidia? Klah-**mee**-dee-ah?
What kind of contraceptive do you use to prevent pregnancy?	¿Qué clase de anticonceptivo usa para prevenir el embarazo? Keh **klah**-seh deh ahn-tee-kohn-sep-**tee**-boh **oo**-sah **pah**-rah preh-beh-**neer** ehl ehm-bah-**rah**-soh?
Condoms?	¿Condones / Preservativos? Kohn-**doh**-nehs / Preh-sehr-bah-**tee**-bohs?
Pills?	¿Pastillas? Pahs-**tee**-yahs?
An intrauterine device?	¿Un dispositivo intrauterino? Oon dees-poh-see-**tee**-boh een-trah-oo-teh-**ree**-noh?
Nothing?	¿Nada? **Nah**-dah?
Have you ever had an ectopic pregnancy?	¿Alguna vez ha tenido un embarazo en un tubo? Ahl-**goo**-nah behs ah teh-**nee**-doh oon ehm-bah-**rah**-soh ehn oon **too**-boh?

Common Phrases for the Exam for Vaginal Bleeding

I am going to examine your abdomen.	Voy a examinarle el abdomen. Boy ah ek-sah-mee-**nahr**-leh ehl ab-**doh**-mehn.

I need to do a rectal exam.	Necesito hacerle un examen del recto. Neh-seh-**see**-toh ah-**sehr**-leh oon ek-**sah**-mehn dehl **rek**-toh.
I need to do a genital exam.	Necesito hacerle un examen genital. Neh-seh-**see**-toh ah-**sehr**-leh oon ek-**sah**-mehn **he**-nee-tahl.
I need to do a pelvic exam.	Necesito hacerle un examen pélvico. Neh-seh-**see**-toh ah-**sehr**-leh oon ek-**sah**-mehn **pehl**-bee-koh.
Bend your knees, please.	Doble las rodillas, por favor. **Doh**-bleh lahs roh-**dee**-yahs, pohr fah-**bohr**.
Separate / Spread your knees, please.	Separe las rodillas, por favor. Seh-**pah**-reh lahs roh-**dee**-yahs, pohr fah-**bohr**.
Do you have pain when I touch here?	¿Tiene dolor cuando le toco aquí? Tee-**eh**-neh doh-**lohr kwahn**-doh leh **toh**-koh ah-**kee**?
We need to do blood and urine tests.	Necesitamos hacerle pruebas de sangre y orina. Neh-seh-see-**tah**-mohs ah-**sehr**-leh **prweh**-bahs deh **sahn**-greh ee oh-**ree**-nah.
We are going to get some X rays.	Vamos a sacarle unas radiografías. **Bah**-mohs ah sah-**kahr**-leh **oo**-nahs rah-dee-oh-grah-**fee**-ahs.

You need an ultrasound.

Usted necesita un ultrasonido.
Oos-**tehd** neh-seh-**see**-tah oon ool-trah-soh-**nee**-doh.

You need an operation.

Usted necesita una operación.
Oos-**tehd** neh-seh-**see**-tah **oo**-nah oh-peh-rah-see-**ohn**.

You are (not) pregnant.

Usted (no) está embarazada.
Oos-**tehd** (noh) ehs-**tah** ehm-bah-rah-**sah**-dah.

You may have a miscarriage or a normal pregnancy.

Puede tener una amenaza de aborto o un embarazo normal.
Pweh-deh teh-**nehr oo**-nah ah-meh-**nah**-sah deh ah-**bohr**-toh oh oon ehm-bah-**rah**-soh nohr-**mahl**.

You have an ectopic pregnancy.

Tiene el embarazo en un tubo.
Tee-**eh**-neh ehl ehm-bah-**rah**-soh ehn oon **too**-boh.

Discharge Instructions for Vaginal Bleeding

Avoid sex, vaginal douching, and tampons.

Evite el sexo, duchas vaginales, y tampones.
Eh-**bee**-teh ehl **sek**-soh, **doo**-chahs bah-hee-**nah**-lehs, ee tahm-**poh**-nehs.

Return in two days to repeat your blood test.

Regrese en dos días para repetir su examen de sangre.
Reh-**greh**-seh ehn dohs **dee**-ahs **pah**-rah reh-peh-**teer** soo ek-**sah**-mehn deh **sahn**-greh.

Return to the hospital (clinic) if . . .

Regrese al hospital (a la clínica) si...
Reh-**greh**-seh ahl ohs-pee-**tahl** (ah lah **klee**-nee-kah) see...

you pass tissue or the bleeding worsens,	pasa tejido / carnosidad o empeora el sangrado, **pah**-sah teh-**hee**-doh / kahr-noh-see-**dahd** oh ehm-peh-**oh**-rah ehl sahn-**grah**-doh,
you have dizziness or headaches,	tiene mareos o dolores de cabeza, tee-**eh**-neh mah-**reh**-ohs oh doh-**loh**-rehs deh kah-**beh**-sah,
you have fever, abdominal pain, or if vomiting continues.	tiene fiebre, dolor abdominal, o si el vómito continúa. tee-**eh**-neh fee-**eh**-breh, doh-**lohr** ab-doh-mee-**nahl**, oh see ehl **boh**-mee-toh kohn-tee-**noo**-ah.

Abdominal Pain in Pregnancy

Dolor Abdominal en el Embarazo

Doh-**lohr** ab-**doh**-mee-nahl ehn ehl ehm-bah-**rah**-soh

Show me where the pain is.	Muéstreme dónde tiene el dolor. **Mwehs**-treh-meh **dohn**-deh tee-**eh**-neh ehl doh-**lohr**.
When did the pain start?	¿Cuándo empezó el dolor? **Kwahn**-doh ehm-peh-**soh** ehl doh-**lohr**?
Is the pain constant?	¿Es el dolor constante? Ehs ehl doh-**lohr** kohns-**tahn**-teh?

Does the pain come and go?	¿El dolor le va y viene? Ehl doh-**lohr** leh bah ee bee-**eh**-neh?
When was your last period?	¿Cuándo fue su última regla / menstruación? **Kwahn**-doh fweh soo **ool**-tee-mah **reh**-glah / mehns-troo-ah-see-**ohn**?
Do you have vaginal bleeding?	¿Tiene sangrado vaginal? Tee-**eh**-neh sahn-**grah**-doh bah-hee-**nahl**?
How many days have you had the bleeding?	¿Por cuántos días ha tenido el sangrado? Pohr **kwahn**-tohs **dee**-ahs ah teh-**nee**-doh ehl sahn-**grah**-doh?
How many pads have you used a day?	¿Cuántas toallas femeninas ha usado al día? **Kwahn**-tahs toh-**ah**-yahs feh-meh-**nee**-nahs ah oo-**sah**-doh ahl **dee**-ah?
Have you passed tissue?	¿Ha pasado carnosidad / tejido? Ah pah-**sah**-doh kahr-noh-see-**dahd** / teh-**hee**-doh?
Do you have a fever?	¿Tiene fiebre? Tee-**eh**-neh fee-**eh**-breh?
Do you have nausea or vomiting?	¿Tiene náusea o vómito? Tee-**eh**-neh **nah**-oo-seh-ah oh **boh**-mee-toh?
Are you urinating more than normal?	¿Orina más de lo normal? Oh-**ree**-nah mahs deh loh nohr-**mahl**?

Do you have burning on urination?	¿Tiene ardor al orinar? Tee-**eh**-neh ahr-**dohr** ahl oh-ree-**nahr**?
Have you received prenatal care?	¿Ha recibido cuidado prenatal? Ah reh-see-**bee**-doh kwih-**dah**-doh preh-nah-**tahl**?
Are you allergic to any medication?	¿Es alérgica a alguna medicina? Ehs ah-**lehr**-hee-kah ah ahl-**goo**-nah meh-dee-**see**-nah?

Common Phrases for the Exam for Abdominal Pain in Pregnancy

I need to do a vaginal exam.	Necesito hacerle un examen vaginal. Neh-seh-**see**-toh ah-**sehr**-leh oon ek-**sah**-mehn bah-hee-**nahl**.
You need an ultrasound.	Usted necesita un ultrasonido. Oos-**tehd** neh-seh-**see**-tah oon ool-trah-soh-**nee**-doh.
I need to do blood and urine tests.	Necesito hacerle pruebas de sangre y orina. Neh-seh-**see**-toh ah-**sehr**-leh **prewh**-bahs deh **sahn**-greh ee oh-**ree**-nah.
You have a urinary tract infection.	Usted tiene una infección de la orina. Oos-**tehd** tee-**eh**-neh **oo**-nah ee-fek-see-**ohn** deh lah oh-**ree**-nah.
You do not have an infection.	Usted no tiene infección. Oos-**tehd** noh tee-**eh**-neh een-fek-see-**ohn**.

You have pain because of stretching of the round ligament of the uterus.	Usted tiene dolor porque se están estirando los ligamentos redondos del útero.
	Oos-**tehd** tee-**eh**-neh doh-**lohr** **pohr**-keh seh ehs-**tahn** ehs-tee-**rahn**-doh lohs lee-gah-**mehn**-tohs reh-**dohn**-dohs dehl **oo**-teh-roh.

Discharge Instructions for Abdominal Pain in Pregnancy

Take your medication.	Tome su medicina.
	Toh-meh soo meh-dee-**see**-nah.
One pill every (X) hours.	Una pastilla cada (X) horas.
	Oo-nah pahs-**tee**-yah **kah**-dah (X) **oh**-rahs.
Return to the hospital (clinic) if you have . . .	Regrese al hospital (a la clínica) si tiene...
	Reh-**greh**-seh ahl ohs-pee-**tahl** (ah lah **klee**-nee-kah) see...
fever,	fiebre,
	fee-**eh**-breh,
vaginal bleeding,	sangrado vaginal,
	sahn-**grah**-doh bah-hee-**nahl**,
or worsening abdominal pain.	o si el dolor abdominal es peor.
	oh see ehl doh-**lohr** ab-doh-mee-**nahl** ehs peh-**ohr**.

Vomiting in Pregnancy	Vómito Durante el Embarazo
	Boh-mee-toh doo-**rahn**-teh ehl ehm-bah-**rah**-soh
When was your last period?	¿Cuándo fue su última regla? **Kwahn**-doh fweh soo **ool**-tee-mah **reh**-glah?
How many times have you been pregnant?	¿Cuántas veces ha estado embarazada? **Kwahn**-tahs **beh**-sehs ah ehs-**tah**-doh ehm-bah-rah-**sah**-dah?
How many children do you have?	¿Cuántos niños tiene? **Kwahn**-tohs **nee**-nyohs tee-**eh**-neh?
When did the vomiting start?	¿Cuándo empezó el vómito? **Kwahn**-doh ehm-peh-**soh** ehl **boh**-mee-toh?
How many times a day do you vomit?	¿Cuántas veces al día vomita? **Kwahn**-tahs **beh**-sehs ahl **dee**-ah boh-**mee**-tah?
When was the last time you vomited?	¿Cuándo fue la última vez que vómito? **Kwahn**-doh fweh lah **ool**-tee-mah behs keh boh-mee-**toh**?
When was the last time you were able to keep something in your stomach?	¿Cuándo fue la última vez que pudo retener algo en el estómago? **Kwahn**-doh fweh lah **ool**-tee-mah behs keh **poo**-doh reh-teh-**nehr ahl**-goh ehn ehl ehs-**toh**-mah-goh?

What color is the emesis?	¿De qué color es el vómito? Deh **keh** koh-**lohr** ehs ehl **boh**-mee-toh?
Is it clear?	¿Es claro? Ehs **klah**-roh?
Is it yellow?	¿Es amarillo? Ehs ah-mah-**ree**-yoh?
Is it green?	¿Es verde? Ehs **behr**-deh?
Is it bloody?	¿Es sangriento? Ehs sahn-gree-**ehn**-toh?
Do you have diarrhea?	¿Tiene diarrea? Tee-**eh**-neh dee-ah-**reh**-ah?
Do you have abdominal pain?	¿Tiene dolor abdominal? Tee-**eh**-neh doh-**lohr** ab-doh-mee-**nahl**?
Do you have vaginal bleeding?	¿Tiene sangrado vaginal? Tee-**eh**-neh sahn-**grah**-doh bah-hee-**nahl**?
Do you have a fever?	¿Tiene fiebre? Tee-**eh**-neh fee-**eh**-breh?
Do you have burning on urination?	¿Tiene ardor al orinar? Tee-**eh**-neh ahr-**dohr** ahl oh-ree-**nahr**?
Are you urinating more than normal?	¿Orina más de lo normal? Oh-**ree**-nah mahs deh loh nohr-**mahl**?
Do you have a cough?	¿Tiene tos? Tee-**eh**-neh tohs?

Common Phrases for the Exam for Vomiting in Pregnancy

You need an IV.	Usted necesita suero intravenoso. Oos-**tehd** neh-seh-**see**-tah soo-**eh**-roh een-trah-beh-**noh**-soh.
You need blood and urine tests.	Usted necesita pruebas de sangre y orina. Oos-**tehd** neh-seh-**see**-tah **prweh**-bahs deh **sahn**-greh ee oh-**ree**-nah.
We need to admit you.	Necesitamos internarla. Neh-seh-see-**tah**-mohs een-tehr-**nahr**-lah.

Discharge Instructions for Vomiting in Pregnancy

Drink only clear liquids (juice).	Tome sólo líquidos claros (jugos). **Toh**-meh **soh**-loh **lee**-kee-dohs **klah**-rohs (**hoo**-gohs).
Eat broth (crackers).	Tome consomés (Coma galletas). **Toh**-meh kohn-soh-**mehs** (**Koh**-mah gah-**yeh**-tahs).
Avoid fried or greasy foods.	Evite las comidas fritas o grasosas. Eh-**bee**-teh lahs koh-**mee**-dahs **free**-tahs oh grah-**soh**-sahs.
Return to the hospital (clinic) if you have . . .	Regrese al hospital (a la clínica) si tiene... Reh-**greh**-seh ahl ohs-pee-**tahl** (ah lah **klee**-nee-kah) see tee-**eh**-neh...

more vomiting,	más vómito, mahs **boh**-mee-toh,
or worsening abdominal pain.	o si el dolor abdominal es peor. oh see ehl doh-**lohr** ab-doh-mee-**nahl** ehs peh-**ohr**.

Labor Pains

Dolores de Parto

Doh-**loh**-rehs deh **pahr**-toh

When did the pain start?	¿Cuándo empezó el dolor? **Kwahn**-doh ehm-peh-**soh** ehl doh-**lohr**?
(X) hours (days) ago.	(X) horas (días). (X) **oh**-rahs (**dee**-ahs).
Do you have pain in your back?	¿Tiene dolor en la espalda? Tee-**eh**-neh doh-**lohr** ehn lah ehs-**pahl**-dah?
Do you have pain in your abdomen?	¿Tiene dolor en el abdomen? Tee-**eh**-neh doh-**lohr** ehn ehl ab-**doh**-mehn?
Are you having contractions?	¿Tiene contracciones? Tee-**eh**-neh kohn-trahk-see- **ohn**-ehs?
Every how many minutes do you get the contractions?	¿Cada cuántos minutos le vienen las contracciones? **Kah**-dah **kwahn**-tohs mee-**noo**- tohs leh bee-**eh**-nehn lahs kohn-trahk-see-**ohn**-ehs?

How many minutes do the contractions last?	¿Cuántos minutos le duran las contracciones? **Kwahn**-tohs mee-**noo**-tohs leh **doo**-rahn lahs kohn-trahk-see-**ohn**-ehs?
Do you have vaginal bleeding?	¿Tiene sangrado vaginal? Tee-**eh**-neh sahn-**grah**-doh bah-hee-**nahl**?
Did your bag of water break?	¿Se le rompió la fuente del agua? Seh leh rohm-pee-**oh** lah **fwehn**-teh dehl **ah**-gwah?
What color was the water?	¿De qué color fue el agua? Deh keh koh-**lohr fweh** ehl **ah**-gwah?
Was it clear?	¿Fue clara? **Fweh klah**-rah?
Was it yellow?	¿Fue amarilla? **Fweh** ah-mah-**ree**-yah?
Was it green?	¿Fue verde? **Fweh behr**-deh?
Was it red?	¿Fue roja? **Fweh roh**-ha?
When did your bag of water break?	¿Cuándo se le reventó la fuente del agua? **Kwahn**-doh seh leh reh-behn-**toh** lah **fwehn**-teh dehl **ah**-gwah?

When was your last period?	¿Cuándo fue su última regla / menstruación? **Kwahn**-doh fweh soo **ool**-tee-mah **reh**-glah / mehns-troo-ah-see-**ohn**?
Month?	¿El mes? Ehl mehs?
Day?	¿El día? Ehl **dee**-ah?
Year?	¿El año? Ehl **ah**-nyoh?
How many pregnancies have you had?	¿Cuántos embarazos ha tenido? **Kwahn**-tohs ehm-bah-**rah**-sohs ah teh-**nee**-doh?
How many children do you have?	¿Cuántos hijos tiene? **Kwahn**-tohs **ee**-hohs tee-**eh**-neh?
Have you received prenatal care?	¿Ha recibido cuidado prenatal? Ah reh-see-**bee**-doh kwi-**dah**-doh preh-nah-**tahl**?
When was the last time you visited your doctor?	¿Cuándo fue la última vez que visitó a su médico? **Kwahn**-doh fweh lah **ool**-tee-mah behs keh bee-see-**toh** ah soo **meh**-dee-koh?
(X) days (weeks, months, years) ago.	(X) días (semanas, meses, años). (X) **dee**-ahs (seh-**mah**-nahs, **meh**-sehs, **ah**-nyohs).

Have you had infections during your pregnancy?	¿Ha tenido infecciones durante su embarazo? Ah teh-**nee**-doh een-fek-see-**ohn**-ehs doo-**rahn**-teh soo ehm-bah-**rah**-soh?
Have you had . . .	¿Ha tenido... Ah teh-**nee**-doh...
gonorrhea?	gonorrea? goh-noh-**reh**-ah?
a urinary (bladder) infection?	una infección urinaria (de la vejiga)? **oo**-nah een-fek-see-**ohn** oo-ree-**nah**-ree-ah (deh lah beh-**hee**-gah)?
syphilis?	sífilis? **see**-fee-lees?
a vaginal infection?	una infección vaginal? **oo**-nah een-fek-see-**ohn** bah-hee-**nahl**?
herpes?	herpes? **ehr**-pehs?
chlamydia?	clamidia? Klah-**mee**-dee-ah?
Did you have problems with your other pregnancies?	¿Ha tenido problemas con los otros embarazos? Ah teh-**nee**-doh proh-**bleh**-mahs kohn lohs **oh**-trohs ehm-bah-**rah**-sohs?
Did you have . . .	¿Tuvo... **Too**-boh...

diabetes?	diabetes? dee-ah-**beh**-tehs?
high blood pressure?	alta presión de la sangre? **ahl**-tah preh-see-**ohn** deh lah **sahn**-greh?
convulsions?	convulsiones? kohn-bool-see-**oh**-nehs?
premature births?	partos prematuros? **pahr**-tohs preh-mah-**too**-rohs?
Did you have babies by vaginal delivery?	¿Tuvo sus bebés por parto vaginal? **Too**-boh soos beh-**behs** pohr **pahr**-toh bah-hee-**nahl**?
Did you have babies by C-section?	¿Tuvo sus bebés por cesárea? **Too**-boh soos beh-**behs** pohr seh-**sah**-reh-ah?

Common Phrases for the Exam for Labor Pains

I need to do a vaginal exam.	Necesito hacerle un examen vaginal. Neh-seh-**see**-toh ah-**sehr**-leh oon ek-**sah**-mehn bah-hee-**nahl**.
(Don't) Push.	(No) Empuje. (Noh) Ehm-**poo**-heh.
You are going to deliver.	Usted va a dar a luz (va a aliviarse). Oos-**tehd** bah ah dahr ah loos (bah ah ah-lee-vee-**ahr**-seh).

I am going to put a monitor on your abdomen.	Voy a ponerle un monitor en el abdomen. **Boh**-ee ah poh-**nehr**-leh oon moh-nee-**tohr** ehn ehl ab-**doh**-mehn.
I am going to listen to the baby's heartbeat.	Voy a escuchar los latidos del corazón del bebé. **Boh**-ee ah ehs-koo-**chahr** lohs lah-**tee**-dohs dehl koh-rah-**sohn** dehl beh-**beh**.
Your cervix is not dilated yet.	Todavía su cuello de la matriz no está dilatado. Toh-dah-**bee**-ah soo **kweh**-yoh deh lah mah-**trees** noh ehs-**tah** dee-lah-**tah**-doh.
You are not in labor yet.	Todavía no va a tener el parto. Toh-dah-**bee**-ah noh bah ah teh-**nehr** ehl **pahr**-toh.
You need an ultrasound to check the baby and the placenta.	Usted necesita un ultrasonido para revisar la condición del bebé y de la placenta. Oos-**tehd** neh-seh-**see**-tah oon ool-trah-soh-**nee**-doh **pah**-rah reh-bee-**sahr** lah kohn-dee-see-**ohn** dehl beh-**beh** ee deh lah plah-**sehn**-tah.

Discharge Instructions for Labor Pains

Return to the hospital (clinic) if . . .	Regrese al hospital (a la clínica) si... Reh-**greh**-seh ahl ohs-pee-**tahl** (ah lah **klee**-nee-kah) see...

your bag of water breaks,	se le rompe la fuente del agua, seh leh **rohm**-peh lah **fwehn**-teh dehl **ah**-gwah,
your pains are more frequent and stronger,	sus dolores son más seguidos y fuertes, soos doh-**loh**-rehs sohn mahs seh-**gee**-dohs ee **fwehr**-tehs,
or you have vaginal bleeding.	o tiene sangrado vaginal. oh tee-**eh**-neh sahn-**grah**-doh bah-hee-**nahl**.

Urinary Tract Infection (UTI)

Infección Urinaria

Een-fek-see-**ohn** oo-ree-**nah**-ree-ah

Does it burn when you urinate?	¿Le arde cuando orina? Leh **ahr**-deh **kwahn**-doh oh-**ree**-nah?
Do you feel pressure over your bladder when you urinate?	¿Siente presión sobre la vejiga cuando orina? See-**ehn**-teh preh-see-**ohn soh**-breh lah beh-**hee**-gah **kwahn**-doh oh-**ree**-nah?
Are you urinating more than normal?	¿Orina más de lo normal? Oh-**ree**-nah mahs deh loh nohr-**mahl**?
Have you noticed blood in your urine?	¿Ha notado sangre en la orina? Ah noh-**tah**-doh **sahn**-greh ehn lah oh-**ree**-nah?

Do you have nausea or vomiting?	¿Tiene náusea o vómito? Tee-**eh**-neh **nah**-oo-seh-ah oh **boh**-mee-toh?
Do you have pain in your side?	¿Tiene dolor en el costado? Tee-**eh**-neh doh-**lohr** ehn ehl kohs-**tah**-doh?
Do you have abdominal pain?	¿Tiene dolor abdominal? Tee-**eh**-neh doh-**lohr** ab-doh-mee-**nahl**?
Do you have a fever?	¿Tiene fiebre? Tee-**eh**-neh fee-**eh**-breh?
Does your urine have a bad odor?	¿Tiene mal olor su orina? Tee-**eh**-neh mahl oh-**lohr** soo oh-**ree**-nah?
Do you have a vaginal discharge?	¿Tiene deshecho vaginal? Tee-**eh**-neh dehs-**eh**-choh bah-hee-**nahl**?
What color is the discharge?	¿De qué color es el deshecho? Deh **keh** koh-**lohr** ehs ehl dehs-**eh**-choh?
Is it yellow?	¿Es amarillo? Ehs ah-mah-**ree**-yoh?
Is it white?	¿Es blanco? Ehs **blahn**-koh?
Is it brown?	¿Es de color café? Ehs deh koh-**lohr** kah-**feh**?
Do you have vaginal itching?	¿Tiene comezón en la vagina? Tee-**eh**-neh koh-meh-**sohn** ehn lah bah-**hee**-nah?

When was your last normal period?

¿Cuándo fue su última regla normal?
Kwahn-doh fweh soo **ool**-tee-mah **reh**-glah nohr-**mahl**?

Are you allergic to penicillin or sulfa?

¿Es alérgica a la penicilina o sulfa?
Ehs ah-**lehr**-hee-kah ah lah peh-nee-see-**lee**-nah oh **sool**-fah?

Do you have . . .

¿Sufre usted de...
Soo-freh oos-**tehd** deh...

    chronic bladder infections?

    infecciones crónicas de la vejiga?
    een-fek-see-**oh**-nehs **kroh**-nee-kahs deh lah beh-**hee**-gah?

    kidney stones?

    cálculos de los riñones?
    kahl-koo-lohs deh lohs ree-**nyoh**-nehs?

    diabetes?

    diabetes?
    dee-ah-**beh**-tehs?

Common Phrases for the Exam for UTI

I need to do a urine test.

Necesito hacerle una prueba de orina.
Neh-seh-**see**-toh ah-**sehr**-leh **oo**-nah **prweh**-bah deh oh-**ree**-nah.

You have a urinary tract infection.

Usted tiene una infección de la orina.
Oos-**tehd** tee-**eh**-neh **oo**-nah een-fek-see-**ohn** deh lah oh-**ree**-nah.

| You need to take antibiotics for the infection. | Necesita tomar antibióticos para la infección.
Neh-seh-**see**-tah toh-**mahr** ahn-tee-bee-**oh**-tee-kohs **pah**-rah lah een-fek-see-**ohn**. |

Discharge Instructions for UTI

| Take the antibiotic every (X) hours. | Tome el antibiótico cada (X) horas.
Toh-meh ehl ahn-tee-bee-**oh**-tee-koh **kah**-dah (X) **oh**-rahs. |

| Drink plenty of liquids. | Tome muchos líquidos.
Toh-meh **moo**-chohs **lee**-kee-dohs. |

| Return to the hospital (clinic) if you have . . . | Regrese al hospital (a la clínica) si tiene...
Reh-**greh**-seh ahl ohs-pee-**tahl** (ah lah **klee**-nee-kah) see tee-**eh**-neh... |

| fever, | fiebre,
fee-**eh**-breh, |

| vomiting, | vómito,
boh-mee-toh, |

| or abdominal pain. | o dolor abdominal.
oh doh-**lohr** ab-doh-mee-**nahl**. |

Rape / Sexual Assault

Violación / Asalto Sexual

Vee-oh-lah-see-**ohn** / Ah-sahl-**toh** sek-soo-ahl

Do you want me to call a friend or relative for you?	¿Quiere que yo le llame a una amistad o pariente? Kee-**eh**-reh keh yoh leh **yah**-meh ah **oo**-nah ah-mees-**tahd** oh pah-ree-**ehn**-teh?
Do you want to speak with . . .	¿Quiere hablar con... Kee-**eh**-reh ab-**blahr** kohn...
a social worker?	un trabajador (una trabajadora) social? oon trah-bah-ha-**dohr** (**oo**-nah trah-bah-hah-**doh**-rah) soh-see-**ahl**?
a psychiatrist?	un / una psiquiatra? oon / **oo**-nah see-kee-**ah**-trah?
the Rape Crisis Center?	el Centro de Crisis para Violaciones? ehl **Sehn**-troh deh **Kree**-sees **pah**-rah Bee-oh-lah-see-**ohn**-ehs?
When did it happen?	¿Cuándo ocurrió? **Kwahn**-doh oh-koo-ree-**oh**?
What time did it happen?	¿A qué hora ocurrió? Ah keh **oh**-rah oh-koo-ree-**oh**?
Do you know who did it?	¿Sabe usted quién lo hizo? **Sah**-beh oos-**tehd** kee-**ehn** loh **ee**-soh?

How many men were there?	¿Cuántos hombres eran? **Kwahn**-tohs **ohm**-brehs **eh**-rahn?
Was there vaginal penetration?	¿Hubo penetración de la vagina? **Oo**-boh peh-neh-trah-see-**ohn** deh lah bah-**hee**-nah?
Was there rectal penetration?	¿Hubo penetración del recto? **Oo**-boh peh-neh-trah-see-**ohn** dehl **rek**-toh?
Was there oral penetration?	¿Hubo penetración oral? **Oo**-boh peh-neh-trah-see-**ohn** oh-**rahl**?
Do you know if the rapist used a condom?	¿Sabe si el violador uso un condón? **Sah**-beh see ehl bee-oh-lah-**dohr** oo-**soh** oon kohn-**dohn**?
Do you know if he ejaculated inside you?	¿Sabe si él eyaculó dentro de usted? **Sah**-beh see ehl eh-yah-koo-**loh dehn**-troh deh oos-**tehd**?
Did he use any foreign objects?	¿Usó él objetos extraños? Oo-**soh** ehl ohb-**heh**-tohs eks-**trah**-nyohs?
Were you beaten?	¿Fue golpeada? Fweh gohl-peh-**ah**-dah?
Were you bitten?	¿Fue mordida? Fweh mohr-**dee**-dah?
Since the rape have you . . .	Desde que fue violada, ¿se ha... **Dehs**-deh keh **fweh** bee-oh-**lah**-dah, seh ah...

showered?	bañado? bah-**nyah**-doh?
changed clothes?	cambiado la ropa? kahm-bee-**ah**-do lah **roh**-pah?
brushed your teeth?	lavado los dientes? lah-**bah**-doh lohs dee-**ehn**-tehs?
urinated?	orinado? oh-ree-**nah**-doh?
defecated?	obrado / defecado? oh-**brah**-doh / deh-feh-**kah**-doh?
When was your last period?	¿Cuándo fue su última regla / menstruación? **Kwahn**-doh fweh soo **ool**-tee-mah **reh**-glah / mehns-troo-ah-see-**ohn**?
Month?	¿El mes? Ehl mehs?
Day?	¿El día? Ehl **dee**-ah?
Year?	¿El año? Ehl **ah**-nyoh?
Are you taking contraceptives?	¿Toma anticonceptivos? **Toh**-mah ahn-tee-kohn-sehp-**tee**-bohs?
When was the last time you had sexual relations?	¿Cuándo fue la última vez que tuvo relaciones sexuales? **Kwahn**-doh fweh lah **ool**-tee-mah behs keh **too**-boh reh-lah-see-**oh**-nehs sek-soo-**ah**-lehs?

Are you allergic to antibiotics?

¿Es alérgica a los antibióticos?
Ehs ah-**lehr**-hee-kah ah lohs
ahn-tee-bee-**oh**-tee-kohs?

Common Phrases for the Exam of the Rape / Sexual Assault Patient

We are going to do a blood and urine test.

Vamos a hacerle una prueba de orina y sangre.
Bah-mohs ah ah-**sehr**-leh **oo**-nah **prweh**-bah deh oh-**ree**-nah ee **sahn**-greh.

We need to collect some cultures.

Necesitamos hacer cultivos.
Neh-seh-see-**tah**-mohs ah-**sehr** kool-**tee**-bohs.

You will receive an injection and pills to prevent venereal diseases.

Recibirá una inyección y pastillas para prevenir enfermedades venéreas.
Reh-see-bee-**rah oo**-nah een-yek-see-**ohn** ee pahs-**tee**-yahs **pah**-rah preh-beh-**neer** ehn-fehr-meh-**dah**-dehs beh-**neh**-reh-ahs.

Would you like me to give you pills to prevent pregnancy?

¿Quiere que le dé pastillas para prevenir el embarazo?
Kee-**eh**-reh keh leh deh pahs-**tee**-yahs **pah**-rah preh-beh-**neer** ehl ehm-bah-**rah**-soh?

Discharge Instructions for Rape / Sexual Assault Patient

Return to the hospital (clinic) if you have . . .

Regrese al hospital (a la clínica) si tiene...
Reh-**greh**-seh ahl ohs-pee-**tahl** (ah lah **klee**-nee-kah) see tee-**eh**-neh...

vaginal bleeding,	sangrado vaginal, sahn-**grah**-doh bah-hee-**nahl**,
vaginal discharge,	deshecho o flujo vaginal, dehs-**eh**-choh oh **floo**-ho bah-hee-**nahl**,
burning on urination,	ardor al orinar, ahr-**dohr** ahl oh-ree-**nahr**,
fever or vomiting,	fiebre o vómito, fee-**eh**-breh oh **boh**-mee-toh,
or severe pain.	o dolor severo (muy fuerte). o doh-**lohr** seh-**beh**-roh (**moo**-ee **fwehr**-teh).

Instructions for the Vitullo Kit

1. I need to comb your hair.

1. Necesito peinarle el pelo.
   Neh-seh-**see**-toh peh-ee-**nahr**-leh ehl **peh**-loh.

2. I need to comb your pubic hair.

2. Necesito peinarle el pelo púbico.
   Neh-seh-**see**-toh peh-see-**nahr**-leh ehl **peh**-loh **poo**-bee-koh.

3. I need to do vaginal cultures.

3. Necesito hacer cultivos vaginales.
   Neh-seh-**see**-toh ah-**sehr** kool-**tee**-bohs bah-hee-**nah**-lehs.

4. I need to get samples from your mouth and rectum.

4. Necesito muestras de su boca y recto.
Neh-seh-**see**-toh **mwehs**-trahs deh soo **boh**-kah ee **rek**-toh.

5. I need to clean under your fingernails.

5. Necesito limpiar debajo de sus uñas.
Neh-seh-**see**-toh leem-pee-**ahr** deh-**bah**-hoh deh soos **oo**-nyahs.

6. Can you leave your underwear for evidence?

6. ¿Puede dejar su ropa interior como evidencia?
Pweh-deh deh-**har** soo **roh**-pah een-teh-ree-**ohr koh**-moh eh-bee-**dehn**-see-ah?

Neurological

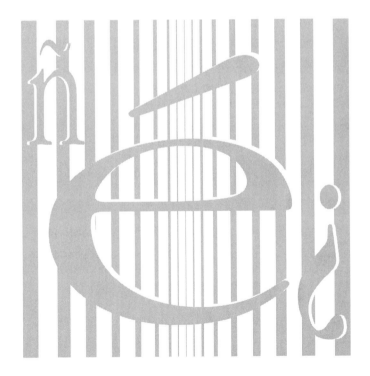

Headache

Dolor de Cabeza

Doh-lohr deh kah-**beh**-sah

Point to where the pain is.

Indique con un dedo dónde tiene el dolor.

Een-**dee**-keh kohn oon **deh**-doh **dohn**-deh tee-**eh**-neh ehl doh-**lohr**.

Do you have pain in your forehead?

¿Tiene dolor en la frente?

Tee-**eh**-neh doh-**lohr** ehn lah **frehn**-teh?

Do you have pain in the back of your head?

¿Tiene dolor en la nuca?

Tee-**eh**-neh doh-**lohr** ehn lah **noo**-kah?

Do you have pain in the neck?

¿Tiene dolor en el cuello?

Tee-**eh**-neh doh-**lohr** ehn ehl **kweh**-yoh?

Does your neck feel stiff or rigid?

¿Siente el cuello tieso o rígido?

See-**ehn**-teh ehl **kweh**-yoh tee-**eh**-soh oh **ree**-hee-doh?

Do you have pain behind the eyes?

¿Siente dolor detras de los ojos?

See-**ehn**-teh doh-**lohr** deh-**trahs** deh lohs **oh**-hohs?

When did the pain start?

¿Cuándo empezó el dolor?

Kwahn-doh ehm-peh-**soh** ehl doh-**lohr**?

(X) hours (days, weeks) ago.

(X) horas (días, semanas).

(X) **oh**-rahs (dee-ahs, seh-**mah**-nahs).

Did the pain start little by little?	¿Empezó el dolor poco a poco? Ehm-peh-**soh** ehl doh-**lohr** **poh**-koh ah **poh**-koh?
Did the pain start all of a sudden?	¿Empezó el dolor de repente? Ehm-peh-**soh** ehl doh-**lohr** deh reh-**pehn**-teh?
Is the pain constant?	¿Es el dolor constante? Ehs ehl doh-**lohr** kohns-**tahn**-teh?
Is the pain intermittent?	¿Es el dolor intermitente? Ehs ehl doh-**lohr** een-tehr-mee-**tehn**-teh?
Is the pain very strong (severe)?	¿Es el dolor muy agudo (severo)? Ehs ehl doh-**lohr moo**-ee ah-**goo**-doh (seh-**beh**-roh)?
Is the pain light?	¿Es el dolor leve? Ehs ehl doh-**lohr** leh-beh?
Is the pain stabbing?	¿Es el dolor punzante? Ehs ehl doh-**lohr** poon-**sahn**-teh?
Do you feel pressure in the head?	¿Siente presión en la cabeza? See-**ehn**-teh preh-see-**ohn** ehn lah kah-**beh**-sah?
Is this the worst headache of your life?	¿Es este el peor dolor de cabeza que ha tenido en su vida? Ehs **ehs**-teh ehl peh-**ohr** doh-**lohr** deh kah-**beh**-sah keh ah teh-**nee**-doh ehn soo **bee**-dah?

Have you ever had this kind of pain before?	¿Ha tenido este tipo de dolor antes? Ah teh-**nee**-doh **ehs**-teh **tee**-poh deh doh-**lohr ahn**-tehs?
When?	¿Cuándo? **Kwahn**-doh?
Do you suffer from migraines?	¿Sufre usted de migrañas / jaquecas? **Soo**-freh oos-**tehd** deh mee-**grah**-nyahs / hah-**keh**-kahs?
Do you have vomiting?	¿Tiene usted vómito? Tee-**eh**-neh oos-**tehd boh**-mee-toh?
Do you have a fever?	¿Tiene fiebre? Tee-**eh**-neh fee-**eh**-breh?
Do you have blurred vision?	¿Tiene la vista borrosa? Tee-**eh**-neh lah **bees**-tah boh-**roh**-sah?
Do you have double vision?	¿Ve usted doble? Beh oos-**tehd doh**-bleh?
Is the pain worse when you look at the light or sun?	¿Le empeora el dolor cuando ve la luz o el sol? Leh ehm-peh-**oh**-rah ehl doh-**lohr kwahn**-doh beh lah loos oh ehl sohl?
Do you feel weak on the left (right) side of your body?	¿Se siente débil en el lado izquierdo (derecho) de su cuerpo? Seh see-**ehn**-teh **deh**-beel ehn ehl **lah**-doh ees-kee-**ehr**-doh (deh-**reh**-choh) deh soo **kwehr**-poh?

| When you have pain, do you have trouble speaking? | Cuando tiene dolor, ¿tiene dificultades para hablar? |
| | **Kwahn**-doh tee-**eh**-neh doh-**lohr**, tee-**eh**-neh dee-fee-kool-**tah**-dehs **pah**-rah ah-**blahr**? |

| Do you have numbness on the left (right) side of your body? | ¿Siente entumido el lado izquierdo (derecho) de su cuerpo? |
| | See-**ehn**-teh ehn-too-**mee**-doh ehl **lah**-doh ees-kee-**ehr**-doh (deh-**reh**-choh) deh soo **kwehr**-poh? |

| Do you have trouble walking? | ¿Tiene dificultades para caminar? |
| | Tee-**eh**-neh dee-fee-kool-**tah**-dehs **pah**-rah kah-mee-**nahr**? |

| Do you have trouble keeping your balance? | ¿Tiene dificultad para mantener su balance? |
| | Tee-**eh**-neh dee-fee-kool-**tahd** **pah**-rah mahn-teh-**nehr** soo bah-**lahn**-seh? |

| Do you wake up with the pain? | ¿Se levanta usted con el dolor? |
| | Seh leh-**bahn**-tah oos-**tehd** kohn ehl doh-**lohr**? |

| Do you get the pain in the middle of the day? | ¿Le da el dolor al mediodía? |
| | Leh dah ehl doh-**lohr** ahl meh-dee-oh-**dee**-ah? |

| Do you get the pain at the end of the afternoon? | ¿Le da el dolor al término de la tarde? |
| | Leh dah ehl doh-**lohr** ahl **tehr**-mee-noh deh lah **tahr**-deh? |

| Do you get the pain at night? | ¿Le da el dolor en la noche? |
| | Leh dah ehl doh-**lohr** ehn lah **noh**-cheh? |

What things give you the pain?

¿Qué cosas le causan dolor?
Keh **koh**-sahs leh **kah**-oo-sahn doh-**lohr**?

Stress in your work (home)?

¿El stress en su trabajo (hogar)?
Ehl ehs-**tres** ehn soo trah-**bah**-hoh (oh-gahr)?

The stress or problems of daily life?

¿El stress o los problemas de la vida diaria?
Ehl ehs-**trehs** oh lohs proh-**bleh**-mahs deh lah **bee**-dah dee-**ah**-ree-ah?

Alcohol?

¿Las bebidas alcohólicas?
Lahs beh-**bee**-dahs ahl-**koh**-lee-kahs?

Family problems?

¿Los problemas familiares?
Lohs proh-**bleh**-mahs fah-mee-lee-**ah**-rehs?

Nothing specific?

¿Nada en particular?
Nah-dah ehn pahr-tee-koo-**lahr**?

Something else?

¿Otra cosa?
Oh-trah **koh**-sah?

What makes the pain better?

¿Qué le mejora el dolor?
Keh leh meh-**hoh**-rah ehl doh-**lohr**?

Did you receive a blow to your head?

¿Recibió usted un golpe a la cabeza?
Reh-see-bee-**oh** oos-**tehd** oon **gohl**-peh ah la kah-**beh**-sah?

Do you suffer from high blood pressure?	¿Padece usted de alta presión de la sangre? Pah-**deh**-seh oos-**tehd** deh **ahl**-tah preh-see-**ohn** deh lah **sahn**-greh?
Do you suffer from diabetes?	¿Padece usted de diabetes? Pah-**deh**-seh oos-**tehd** deh dee-ah-**beh**-tehs?
Do you drink alcohol?	¿Toma usted bebidas alcohólicas? Toh-mah oos-tehd beh-**bee**-dahs ahl-**koh**-lee-kahs?
Do you use drugs?	¿Usa drogas? **Oo**-sah **droh**-gahs?
Do you use marihuana (cocaine, heroin)?	¿Usa marijuana (cocaína, heroína)? **Oo**-sah mah-ree-**hwah**-nah (koh-kah-**ee**-nah, eh-roh-**ee**-nah)?

Common Phrases for the Exam for Headache

You need a CT scan of the brain.	Usted necesita un CT / una tomografía del cerebro. Oos-**tehd** neh-seh-**see**-tah oon **seh**-teh / **oo**-nah toh-moh-grah-**fee**-ah dehl seh-**reh**-broh.
We are going to give you an injection for the pain.	Vamos a darle una inyección para el dolor. **Bah**-mohs ah **dahr**-leh **oo**-nah een-jeg-see-**ohn pah**-rah ehl doh-**lohr**.

I am going to give you a pill for the pain.

Voy a darle una pastilla para el dolor.
Boh-ee ah **dahr**-leh **oo**-nah pahs-**tee**-yah **pah**-rah ehl doh-**lohr**.

You have a headache because of nervous tension.

Usted tiene dolor de cabeza por tensión nerviosa.
Oos-**tehd** tee-**eh**-neh doh-**lohr** deh kah-**beh**-sah pohr tehn-see-**ohn** nehr-bee-**oh**-sah.

You have migraines.

Usted sufre de migrañas / jaquecas.
Oos-**tehd** soo-freh deh mee-**grah**-nyahs / hah-**keh**-kahs.

You have meningitis (an infection of the brain).

Usted tiene meningitis (infección en el cerebro).
Oos-**tehd** tee-**eh**-neh meh-neen-**hee**-tees (een-fek-see-**ohn** ehn ehl seh-**reh**-broh).

You have a cerebral hemorrhage (bleeding in your brain).

Usted tiene una hemorragia cerebral (un sangrado en el cerebro).
Oos-**tehd** tee-**eh**-neh **oo**-nah eh-moh-**rah**-hee-ah seh-reh-**brahl** (oon sahn-**grah**-doh ehn ehl se-**reh**-broh).

You have a tumor.

Usted tiene un tumor.
Oos-**tehd** tee-**eh**-neh oon too-**mohr**.

You had a stroke.

Usted tuvo una embolia.
Oos-**tehd too**-boh **oo**-nah ehm-**boh**-lee-ah.

Neurologic Exam for Headache

What is your name?
¿Cuál es su nombre?
Kwahl ehs soo **nohm**-breh?

or ¿Cómo se llama?
Koh-moh seh **yah**-mah?

What is the date today?
¿Cuál es la fecha hoy?
Kwahl ehs lah **feh**-chah **oh**-ee?

Do you know where you are now?
¿Sabe dónde está en este momento?
Sah-beh **dohn**-deh ehs-**tah** ehn **ehs**-teh moh-**mehn**-toh?

What is your birth date?
¿Cuál es la fecha de su nacimiento?
Kwahl ehs lah **feh**-chah deh soo nah-see-mee-**ehn**-toh?

What is your phone number?
¿Cuál es su número de teléfono?
Kwahl ehs soo **noo**-meh-roh deh teh-**leh**-foh-noh?

Squeeze my hand hard.
Apriete mi mano fuerte.
Ah-pree-**eh**-teh mee **mah**-noh **fwehr**-teh.

Pull me toward you.
Jáleme hacia usted.
Ha-leh-meh **ah**-see-ah oos-**tehd**.

Raise your leg.
Levante la pierna.
Leh-**bahn**-teh lah pee-**ehr**-nah.

Walk a straight line.
Camine en una línea recta.
Kah-**mee**-neh ehn **oo**-nah **lee**-neh-ah **rehk**-tah.

Smile.	Sonría. Sohn-**ree**-ah.
Show me your teeth.	Muéstreme los dientes. **Mwehs**-treh-meh lohs dee-**ehn**-tehs.
Close both eyes.	Cierre ambos ojos. See-**eh**-reh **ahm**-bohs **oh**-hos.
Do you feel me touching you?	¿Siente que lo / la estoy tocando? See-**ehn**-teh keh loh / lah ehs-**toy** toh-**kahn**-doh?

Instructions for Lumbar Puncture

I need to do a special test to see if you have meningitis (an infection in the brain).	Necesito hacerle un examen especial para ver si tiene meningitis (una infección en el cerebro). Neh-seh-**see**-toh ah-**sehr**-leh oon ek-**sah**-mehn ehs-peh-see-**ahl pah**-rah behr see tee-**eh**-neh meh-neen-**hee**-tees (**oo**-nah een-fek-see-**ohn** ehn ehl seh-**reh**-broh).
I am going to put a needle in your back to draw some fluid that surrounds the brain.	Voy a ponerle una aguja en la espalda para sacarle líquido que rodea al cerebro. **Boh**-ee ah poh-**nehr**-leh **oo**-nah ah-**goo**-hah ehn lah ehs-**pahl**-dah **pah**-rah sah-**kahr**-leh **lee**-kee-doh keh roh-**deh**-ah ahl seh-**reh**-broh.
I need to do a lumbar puncture.	Necesito hacerle una punción lumbar. Neh-seh-**see**-toh ah-**sehr**-leh **oo**-nah poon-see-**ohn** loom-**bahr.**

Stay on your right (left) side and bend your knees up toward your chest.	Póngase de lado derecho (izquierdo) y doble las rodillas hacia el pecho. **Pohn**-gah-seh dehl **lah**-doh deh-**reh**-choh (ees-kee-**ehr**-doh) ee **doh**-bleh lahs roh-**dee**-yahs **ah**-see-ah ehl **peh**-choh.
Don't move during this exam.	No se mueva durante este examen. Noh seh **mweh**-bah doo-**rahn**-teh **ehs**-teh ek-**sah**-mehn.
After the lumbar puncture . . .	Después de la punción lumbar... Dehs-**pwehs** deh lah poon-see-**ohn** loom-**bahr**...
Lie on your back.	Acuéstese boca arriba. Ah-**kwehs**-teh-seh **boh**-kah ah-**ree**-bah.
You need to lie on your back for 2 hours.	Necesita acostarse boca arriba por dos horas. Neh-seh-**see**-tah ah-kohs-**tar**-seh **boh**-kah ah-**ree**-bah pohr dohs **oh**-ras.
Tell me if your headache worsens.	Dime si el dolor se pone peor. **Dee**-meh see ehl doh-**lohr** seh **poh**-neh peh-**ohr**.

Discharge Instructions for Headache

Take your medicine.	Tome su medicina. **Toh**-me soo meh-dee-**see**-nah.
Return to the hospital (clinic) if . . .	Regrese al hospital (a la clínica) si... Reh-**greh**-seh ahl ohs-pee-**tahl** (ah lah **klee**-nee-kah) see...

the headache worsens,	el dolor de cabeza empeora, ehl doh-**lohr** deh kah-**beh**-sah ehm-peh-**oh**-rah,
your neck becomes stiff,	su cuello se pone rígido / tieso, soo **kweh**-yoh seh **poh**-neh **ree**-hee-doh / tee-**eh**-soh,
you have fever, vomiting, or problems with your balance.	tiene fiebre, vómito, o problemas con su balance. tee-**eh**-neh fee-**eh**-breh, **boh**-mee-toh, oh proh-**bleh**-mahs kohn soo bah-**lahn**-seh.

Dizziness — Mareos

Mah-**reh**-ohs

How long have you been dizzy?	¿Por cuánto tiempo ha estado mareado / -a? Pohr **kwahn**-toh tee-**ehm**-poh ah ehs-**tah**-doh mah-reh-**ah**-doh / -dah?
For (X) hours (days, weeks, months).	Desde (X) horas (días, semanas, meses). **Dehz**-deh (X) **oh**-ras (dee-ahs, seh-**mah**-nahs, **meh**-ses).
Do you feel the room spinning?	¿Siente que el cuarto le da vueltas? See-**ehn**-teh keh ehl **kwahr**-toh leh dah **bwehl**-tahs?

Do you feel yourself spinning around the room?	¿Siente que usted da vueltas alrededor del cuarto? See-**ehn**-teh keh oos-**tehd** dah **bwehl**-tahs ahl-reh-deh-**dohr** dehl **kwahr**-toh?
Have you felt any other symptoms?	¿Ha sentido algún otro síntoma? Ah sehn-**tee**-doh ahl-**goon oh**-troh **seen**-toh-mah?
Deafness?	¿Sordera? Sohr-**deh**-rah?
Ringing in the ears?	¿Zumbido en los oídos? Soom-**bee**-doh ehn lohs oh-**ee**-dohs?
Earache?	¿Dolor de oído? Doh-**lohr** deh oh-**ee**-doh?
Pus from your ear?	¿Pus del oído? Poos dehl oh-**ee**-doh?
Palpitations?	¿Palpitaciones? Pahl-pee-tah-see-**oh**-nehs?
Chest pain?	¿Dolor en el pecho? Doh-**lohr** ehn ehl **peh**-choh?
Numbness (tingling) in your hands or feet?	¿Entumido (hormigueo) en las manos o pies? Ehn-too-**mee**-doh (ohr-mee-**geh**-oh) ehn lahs **mah**-nohs oh pee-**ehs**?
Vomiting?	¿Vómito? **Boh**-mee-toh?

Problems with your balance?	¿Problemas con su balance? Proh-**bleh**-mahs kohn soo bah-**lahn**-seh?
Are you dizzy when you sit still?	¿Siente mareos cuando esta quieto / -a? See-**ehn**-teh mah-**reh**-ohs **kwahn**-doh ehs-**tah** kee-**eh**-toh / -tah?
Do you feel dizzy when you move your head?	¿Se siente mareado / -a cuando mueve la cabeza? Seh see-**ehn**-teh mah-reh-**ah**-doh / -dah **kwahn**-doh **mweh**-beh lah kah-**beh**-sah?
Are you dizzy when you stand up?	¿Se siente mareado / -a cuando se levanta (se para)? Seh see-**ehn**-teh mah-reh-**ah**-doh / -dah **kwahn**-doh seh leh-**bahn**-tah (seh **par**-rah)?
Is the dizziness better (worse, the same) since it started?	¿Son los mareos mejores (peores, iguales) desde que empezaron? Sohn lohs mah-**reh**-ohs meh-**hoh**-rehs (peh-**oh**-rehs, ee-**gwah**-lehs) **dehs**-deh keh ehm-peh-**sah**-rohn?
Have you had a cold recently?	¿Recientemente ha tenido usted un resfriado? Reh-see-ehn-teh-**mehn**-teh ah teh-**nee**-doh oos-**tehd** oon rehs-free-**ah**-doh?
Did you hit your head recently?	¿Recientemente se pegó en la cabeza? Reh-see-ehn-teh-**mehn**-teh seh peh-**goh** ehn lah kah-**beh**-sah?

Do you have . . .	Sufre usted de... **Soo**-freh oos-**tehd** deh...
high blood pressure?	alta presión de la sangre? **ahl**-tah preh-see-**ohn** deh lah **sahn**-greh?
diabetes?	diabetes? dee-ah-**beh**-tehs?
heart disease?	enfermedad del corazón? ehn-fehr-meh-**dad** dehl koh-rah-**sohn**?
Are you taking any medications?	¿Toma algún medicamento? **Toh**-mah ahl-**goon** meh-dee-kah-**mehn**-toh?
What are you taking?	¿Qué toma? Keh **toh**-mah?

Common Phrases for the Exam for Dizziness

We are going to do an EKG.	Vamos a hacerle un electrocardiograma. **Bah**-mohs ah ah-**sehr**-leh oon eh-lek-troh-kar-dee-oh-**grah**-mah.
We are going to do some blood tests.	Vamos a hacerle unas pruebas de sangre. **Bah**-mohs ah ah-**sehr**-leh **oo**-nahs **prweh**-bahs deh **sahn**-greh.
You need an X ray (CT scan) of your head.	Usted necesita una radiografía (tomografía) de la cabeza. Oos-**tehd** neh-seh-**see**-tah **oo**-nah rah-dee-oh-grah-**fee**-ah (toh-moh-grah-**fee**-ah) deh lah kah-**beh**-sah.

Lie down (Sit up, Stand up) so I can take your blood pressure.

Acuéstese (Siéntese, Párese) para que pueda tomarle la presión de la sangre.
Ah-**kwehs**-teh-seh (See-**ehn**-teh-seh, **Pah**-reh-seh) **pah**-rah keh **pweh**-dah toh-**mahr**-leh lah preh-see-**ohn** deh lah **sahn**-greh.

I need to do a rectal exam.

Necesito hacerle un examen del recto.
Neh-seh-**see**-toh ah-**sehr**-leh oon ek-**sah**-mehn dehl **rek**-toh.

You had a stroke.

Usted tuvo una embolia.
Oos-**tehd too**-boh **oo**-nah ehm-**boh**-lee-ah.

You have a cerebral hemorrhage (bleeding in your brain).

Usted tiene una hemorragia cerebral (un sangrado en el cerebro).
Oos-**tehd** tee-**eh**-neh **oo**-nah eh-moh-**rah**-hee-ah seh-reh-**brahl** (oon sahn-**grah**-doh ehn ehl seh-**reh**-broh).

You have problems with your inner ear.

Usted tiene problemas con su oído interno.
Oos-**tehd** tee-**eh**-neh proh-**bleh**-mahs kohn soo oh-**ee**-doh een-**tehr**-noh.

Neurologic Exam for Dizziness

What is your name?

¿Cuál es su nombre?
Kwahl ehs soo **nohm**-breh?

or ¿Cómo se llama?
Koh-moh seh **yah**-mah?

What is the date today?	¿Cuál es la fecha de hoy? Kwahl ehs lah **feh**-chah deh **oh**-ee?
Do you know where you are now?	¿Sabe dónde está en este momento? **Sah**-beh **dohn**-deh ehs-**tah** ehn **ehs**-teh moh-**mehn**-toh?
What is your birth date?	¿Cuál es la fecha de su nacimiento? Kwahl ehs lah **feh**-chah deh soo nah-see-mee-**ehn**-toh?
What is your phone number?	¿Cuál es su número de teléfono? Kwahl ehs soo **noo**-meh-roh deh teh-**leh**-foh-noh?
Squeeze my hand hard.	Apriete mi mano fuerte. Ah-pree-**eh**-teh mee **mah**-noh **fwehr**-teh.
Pull me toward you.	Jáleme hacia usted. **Ha**-leh-meh **ah**-see-ah oos-**tehd.**
Raise your leg.	Levante la pierna. Leh-**bahn**-teh lah pee-**ehr**-nah.
Walk a straight line.	Camine en una línea recta. Kah-**mee**-neh ehn **oo**-nah **lee**-neh-ah **rehk**-tah.
Smile.	Sonría. Sohn-**ree**-ah.
Show me your teeth.	Muéstreme los dientes. **Mwehs**-treh-meh lohs dee-**ehn**-tehs.
Close both eyes.	Cierre ambos ojos. See-**eh**-reh **ahm**-bohs **oh**-hos.

Do you feel me touching you?	¿Siente que lo / la estoy tocando? See-**ehn**-teh keh loh / lah ehs-**toy** toh-**kahn**-doh?

Discharge Instructions for Dizziness

Take the medicine (X) times a day.	Tome la medicina (X) veces al día. **Toh**-meh lah meh-dee-**see**-nah (X) **beh**-sehs ahl **dee**-ah.
Return to the hospital (clinic) if . . .	Regrese al hospital (a la clínica) si... Reh-**greh**-seh ahl ohs-pee-**tahl** (ah lah **klee**-nee-kah) see...
your dizziness is worse,	sus mareos son peores, soos mah-**reh**-ohs sohn peh-**oh**-rehs,
you have vomiting,	tiene vómito, tee-**eh**-neh **boh**-mee-toh,
you feel numbness or weakness in your arms or legs.	siente entumidos o débiles los brazos o piernas. see-**ehn**-teh ehn-too-**mee**-dohs oh **deh**-bee-lehs lohs **brah**-sohs oh pee-**ehr**-nahs.

Syncope

Desmayo

Dehs-mah-**yoh**

When did you faint?	¿Cuándo se desmayó? **Kwahn**-doh seh dehs-mah-**yoh**?

(X) minutes (hours, days) ago.	(X) minutos (horas, días). (X) mee-**noo**-tohs (**oh**-rahs, **dee**-ahs).
Did you lose consciousness when you fainted?	¿Perdió el conocimiento cuando se desmayó? Pehr-dee-**oh** ehl koh-noh-see-mee-**ehn**-toh **kwahn**-doh seh dehs-mah-**yoh**?
How long were you unconscious?	¿Por cuánto tiempo estuvo inconciente? Pohr **kwahn**-toh tee-**ehm**-poh ehs-**too**-boh een-kohn-see-**ehn**-teh?
(X) minutes (hours).	(X) minutos (horas). (X) mee-**noo**-tohs (**oh**-rahs).
What were you doing when you fainted?	¿Qué estaba haciendo cuándo se desmayó? Keh ehs-**tah**-bah ah-see-**ehn**-doh **kwahn**-doh seh dehs-mah-**yoh**?
Were you sitting?	¿Estaba sentado / -a? Ehs-**tah**-bah sehn-**tah**-doh / -dah?
Were you lying down?	¿Estaba acostado / -a? Ehs-**tah**-bah ah-kohs-**tah**-doh / -dah?
Were you walking?	¿Estaba caminando? Ehs-**tah**-bah kah-mee-**nahn**-doh?
Were you standing?	¿Estaba parado / -a? Ehs-**tah**-bah pah-**rah**-doh / -dah?

Were you urinating?

¿Estaba orinando?
Ehs-**tah**-bah oh-ree-**nahn**-doh?

Were you defecating?

¿Estaba defecando /
obrando?
Ehs-**tah**-bah deh-feh-**kahn**-doh / oh-**brahn**-doh?

Did you faint after . . .

¿Se desmayó después de...
Seh dehs-mah-**yoh** dehs-**pwehs** deh...

getting out of bed?

levantarse de la cama?
leh-bahn-**tahr**-seh deh lah
kah-mah?

emotional upset?

algún enojo emocional?
ahl-**goon** eh-**noh**-ho eh-moh-see-oh-**nahl**?

hitting yourself in the
head?

pegarse en la cabeza?
peh-**gahr**-seh ehn lah kah-**beh**-sah?

Before you fainted, did
you . . .

Antes de desmayarse,...
Ahn-tehs deh dehs-mah-**yahr**-seh...

have chest pain?

¿tuvo dolor del pecho?
too-boh doh-**lohr** dehl
peh-choh?

have chest pressure?

¿tuvo presión en el
pecho?
too-boh preh-see-**ohn** ehn
ehl **peh**-choh?

have sweating?

¿tuvo sudor?
too-boh soo-**dohr**?

have palpitations?	¿tuvo palpitaciones? **too**-boh pahl-pee-tah-see-**oh**-nehs?
have shortness of breath?	¿tuvo falta de aire? **too**-boh **fahl**-tah deh ah-ee-reh?
have a headache?	¿tuvo dolor de cabeza? **too**-boh doh-**lohr** deh kah-**beh**-sah?
have abdominal pain?	¿tuvo dolor abdominal? **too**-boh doh-**lohr** ab-doh-mee-**nahl**?
have blurred vision?	¿tuvo la vista borrosa? **too**-boh lah **bees**-tah boh-**roh**-sah?
feel hot and nauseous?	¿sintió calor y náusea? seen-tee-**oh** kah-**lohr** ee **nah**-oo-seh-ah?
How many times did you faint today?	¿Cuántas veces se desmayó hoy? **Kwahn**-tahs **beh**-sehs seh dehs-mah-**yoh oh**-ee?
Have you fainted before?	¿Se ha desmayado antes? Seh ah dehs-mah-**yah**-doh **ahn**-tehs?
Have you had vomiting?	¿Ha tenido vómito? Ah teh-**nee**-doh **boh**-mee-toh?
Have you vomited blood?	¿Ha vomitado sangre? Ah boh-mee-**tah**-doh **sahn**-greh?
Have you had rectal bleeding?	¿Ha tenido sangrado rectal? Ah teh-**nee**-doh sahn-**grah**-doh rek-**tahl**?

Have you noticed black stools?	¿Ha notado heces negras? Ah noh-**tah**-doh **eh**-sehs **neh**-grahs?
Did you have a seizure?	¿Tuvo un ataque epiléptico? **Too**-boh oon ah-**tah**-keh eh-pee-**lep**-tee-koh?
Did you lose control of your bladder?	¿Perdió control de la orina? Pehr-dee-**oh** kohn-**trohl** deh lah oh-**ree**-nah?
Did you bite your tongue?	¿Se mordió la lengua? Seh mohr-dee-**oh** lah **lehn**-gwah?
Do you have chest pain now?	¿Tiene dolor del pecho ahora? Tee-**eh**-neh doh-**lohr** dehl **peh**-choh ah-**oh**-rah?
Do you have a headache now?	¿Tiene dolor de cabeza ahora? Tee-**eh**-neh doh-**lohr** deh kah-**beh**-sah ah-**oh**-rah?
Do you have weakness in any part of your body?	¿Tiene debilidad en alguna parte del cuerpo? Tee-**eh**-neh deh-bee-lee-**dahd** ehn ahl-**goo**-nah **pahr**-teh dehl **kwehr**-poh?
Do you have numbness in any part of your body?	¿Tiene entumida alguna parte del cuerpo? Tee-**eh**-neh ehn-too-**mee**-dah ahl-**goo**-nah **pahr**-teh dehl **kwehr**-poh?
Show me where you have weakness (numbness).	Muéstreme dónde tiene debilidad (entumecimiento). **Muehs**-treh-meh **dohn**-deh tee-**eh**-neh deh-bee-lee-**dahd** (ehn-too-meh-see-mee-**ehn**-toh).

Do you have trouble talking?	¿Tiene problemas para hablar? Tee-**eh**-neh proh-**bleh**-mahs **pah**-rah ah-**blahr**?
Do you suffer from heart disease?	¿Sufre de enfermedades del corazón? **Soo**-freh deh ehn-fehr-meh-**dah**-dehs dehl koh-rah-**sohn**?
Have you ever had a stroke?	¿Alguna vez ha tenido una embolia? Ahl-**goo**-nah behs ah teh-**nee**-doh **oo**-nah ehm-**boh**-lee-ah?
Do you have a pacemaker?	¿Tiene un marcapaso? Tee-**eh**-neh oon mahr-kah-**pah**-soh?
When was your pacemaker last checked?	¿Cuándo fue la última vez que le chequearon (revisaron) el marcapaso? **Kwahn**-doh fweh lah **ool**-tee-mah behs keh leh cheh-keh-**ah**-rohn (reh-bee-**sah**-rohn) ehl **mahr**-kah-**pah**-soh?

Common Phrases for the Exam for Syncope

You need an EKG.	Usted necesita un electrocardiograma. Oos-**tehd** neh-seh-**see**-tah oon eh-lek-troh-kahr-dee-oh-**grah**-mah.
You need to get a CT scan of your head.	Usted necesita una radiografía (una tomografía) de la cabeza. Oos-**tehd** neh-seh-**see**-tah **oo**-nah rah-dee-oh-grah-**fee**-ah (**oo**-nah toh-moh-grah-**fee**-ah) deh lah kah-**beh**-sah.

You have low blood pressure.

Usted tiene baja la presión de la sangre.
Oos-**tehd** tee-**eh**-neh **bah**-hah lah preh-see-**ohn** deh lah **sahn**-greh.

You have a heart blockage.

Usted tiene un bloqueo del corazón.
Oos-**tehd** tee-**eh**-neh oon bloh-**keh**-oh dehl koh-rah-**sohn**.

You have a low pulse.

Usted tiene el pulso bajo.
Oos-**tehd** tee-**eh**-neh ehl **pool**-soh **bah**-hoh.

You had a stroke.

Usted tuvo una embolia.
Oos-**tehd too**-boh **oo**-nah ehm-**boh**-lee-ah.

We are going to take your blood pressure lying and standing.

Vamos a tomarle la presión acostado / -a y parado / -a.
Bah-mohs ah toh-**mahr**-leh lah preh-see-**ohn** ah-kohs-**tah**-doh / -dah ee pah-**rah**-doh / -dah.

We are going to take your pulse lying and standing.

Vamos a tomarle el pulso acostado / -a y parado / -a.
Bah-mohs ah toh-**mahr**-leh ehl **pool**-soh ah-kohs-**tah**-doh / -dah ee pah-**rah**-doh / -dah.

Tell me if you feel dizzy when you stand up.

Dígame si se siente mareado / -a cuando se para.
Dee-gah-meh see seh see-**ehn**-teh mah-reh-**ah**-doh / -dah **kwahn**-doh seh **pah**-rah.

I need to do a rectal exam.

Necesito hacerle un examen rectal.
Neh-seh-**see**-toh ah-**sehr**-leh oon ek-**sah**-mehn rek-**tahl**.

You need an IV.	Usted necesita suero intravenoso. Oos-**tehd** neh-seh-**see**-tah soo-**eh**-roh een-trah-beh-**noh**-soh.
You need a blood transfusion.	Usted necesita una transfusión de sangre. Oos-**tehd** neh-seh-**see**-tah **oo**-nah trahns-foo-see-**ohn** deh **sahn**-greh.
You need a pacemaker.	Usted necesita un marcapaso. Oos-**tehd** neh-seh-**see**-tah oon **mahr**-kah-**pah**-soh.
You fainted because you got up too fast.	Se desmayó porque se paró muy rápido. Seh dehs-mah-**yoh pohr**-keh seh pah-**roh moo**-ee **rah**-pee-doh.

Discharge Instructions for Syncope

Sit by the side of the bed for two minutes before getting up.	Siéntese al lado de la cama por dos minutos antes de pararse. See-**ehn**-teh-seh ahl **lah**-doh deh lah **kah**-mah pohr dohs mee-**noo**-tohs **ahn**-tehs deh pah-**rahr**-seh.
Return to the hospital (clinic) if . . .	Regrese al hospital (a la clínica) si... Reh-**greh**-seh ahl ohs-pee-**tahl** (ah lah **klee**-nee-kah) see...
you keep fainting,	sigue desmayándose, **see**-geh dehs-mah-**yahn**-doh-seh,

you have chest pain,	tiene dolor del pecho, tee-**eh**-neh doh-**lohr** dehl **peh**-choh,
or you have dizziness.	o tiene mareos. oh tee-**eh**-neh mah-**reh**- ohs.

Stroke

Embolia o Derrame Cerebral

Ehm-**boh**-lee-ah oh deh-**rah**-meh seh-reh-**brahl**

When did the stroke occur?	¿Cuándo ocurrió la embolia? **Kwahn**-doh oh-koo-ree-**oh** lah ehm-**boh**-lee-ah?
(X) hours (days, weeks) ago.	(X) horas (días, semanas). (X) **oh**-rahs (**dee**-ahs, seh- **mah**-nahs).
Did he / she / you wake up with the stroke?	¿Se despertó con la embolia? Seh dehs-pehr-**toh** kohn lah ehm-**boh**-lee-ah?
What part of his / her / your body is weak (numb)?	¿Qué parte del cuerpo está débil (entumida)? Keh **pahr**-teh dehl **kwehr**-poh ehs-tah deh-beel (ehn-too- **mee**-dah)?
His / Her / Your face?	¿La cara? Lah **kah**-rah?
His / Her / Your right (left) arm?	¿El brazo derecho (izquierdo)? Ehl **brah**-soh deh-**reh**-choh (ees-kee-**ehr**-doh)?

His / Her / Your right (left) leg?

¿La pierna derecha (izquierda)?
Lah pee-**ehr**-nah deh-**reh**-chah (ees-kee-**ehr**-dah)?

His / Her / Your right (left) side?

¿El lado derecho (izquierdo)?
Ehl **lah**-doh deh-**reh**-choh (ees-kee-**ehr**-doh)?

Does he / she (Do you) have difficulty speaking?

¿Tiene dificultad para hablar?
Tee-**eh**-neh dee-fee-kool-**tahd pah**-rah ah-**blahr**?

Does he / she (Do you) have trouble understanding written (spoken) words?

¿Tiene problemas al entender palabras escritas (habladas)?
Tee-**eh**-neh proh-**bleh**-mahs ahl ehn-tehn-**dehr** pah-**lah**-brahs ehs-**kree**-tahs (ah-**blah**-dahs)?

Did he / she / you fall?

¿Se cayó?
Seh kah-**yoh**?

Does he / she (Do you) have trouble walking?

¿Tiene problemas al caminar?
Tee-**eh**-neh proh-**bleh**-mahs ahl kah-mee-**nahr**?

Can he / she / you walk?

¿Puede caminar?
Pweh-deh kah-mee-**nahr**?

Does he / she (Do you) have trouble keeping his / her / your balance?

¿Tiene problemas para mantener su balance?
Tee-**eh**-neh proh-**bleh**-mahs **pah**-rah mahn-teh-**nehr** soo bah-**lahn**-seh?

Has he / she (Have you) complained of a headache?

¿Se ha quejado de dolor de cabeza?
Seh ah keh-**ha**-doh deh doh-**lohr** deh kah-**beh**-sah?

Has he / she (Have you) complained of dizzy spells?

¿Se ha quejado de mareos?
Seh ah keh-**ha**-doh deh mah-**reh**-ohs?

Is this his / her / your first stroke?

¿Es ésta su primera embolia?
Ehs **ehs**-tah soo pree-**meh**-rah ehm-**boh**-lee-ah?

Does he / she (Do you) have hypertension?

¿Tiene alta presión de la sangre?
Tee-**eh**-neh **ahl**-tah preh-see-**ohn** deh lah **sahn**-greh?

Does he / she (Do you) have heart problems?

¿Tiene problemas del corazón?
Tee-**eh**-neh proh-**bleh**-mahs dehl koh-rah-**sohn**?

Does he / she (Do you) have diabetes?

¿Tiene diabetes?
Tee-**eh**-neh dee-ah-**beh**-tehs?

Does he / she (Do you) have Parkinson's disease?

¿Tiene enfermedad de Párkinson?
Tee-**eh**-neh ehn-fehr-meh-**dahd** deh **pahr**-keen-sohn?

Does he / she (Do you) have epilepsy?

¿Tiene epilepsia?
Tee-**eh**-neh eh-pee-**lep**-see-ah?

Does he / she (Do you) have multiple sclerosis?

¿Tiene esclerosis múltiple?
Tee-**eh**-neh ehs-kleh-**roh**-sees **mool**-tee-pleh?

Is he / she (Are you) on blood thinners?

¿Toma medicina para adelgazarle la sangre?
Toh-mah meh-dee-**see**-nah **pah**-rah ah-dehl-gah-**sahr**-leh lah **sahn**-greh?

Common Phrases for the Exam for Stroke

He / She needs (You need) a CT scan.	Necesita una radiografía de la cabeza. Neh-seh-**see**-tah **oo**-nah rah-dee-oh-grah-**fee**-ah deh lah kah-**beh**-sah.
He / She has (You have) had a stroke.	Ha tenido una embolia. Ah teh-**nee**-doh **oo**-nah ehm-**boh**-lee-ah.
He / She / You had a TIA.	Tuvo un ataque de isquemia transitorio. **Too**-boh oon ah-**tah**-keh deh ees-**keh**-mee-ah trahn-see-**toh**-ree-oh.
He / She has (You have) a cerebral hemorrhage.	Tiene un derrame cerebral. Tee-**eh**-neh oon deh-**rah**-meh seh-reh-**brahl**.
He / She needs (You need) to see a neurologist.	Necesita ver a un neurólogo. Neh-seh-**see**-tah behr ah oon neh-oo-**roh**-loh-goh.
He / She needs (You need) to see a neurosurgeon.	Necesita ver a un neurocirujano. Neh-seh-**see**-tah behr ah oon **neh**-oo-roh-see-roo-**hah**-noh.

# Seizures	# Convulsiones
	Kohn-vool-**see**-oh-nehs
When did it happen?	¿Cuándo ocurrio? **Kwahn**-doh oh-koo-ree-**oh**?

(X) hours (days, weeks) ago.

(X) horas (días, semanas).
(X) **oh**-rahs (**dee**-ahs, seh-**mah**-nahs).

How long did the attack last?

¿Cuánto tiempo duró el ataque?
Kwahn-toh tee-**ehm**-poh doo-**roh** ehl ah-**tah**-keh?

(X) seconds (minutes).

(X) segundos (minutos).
(X) seh-**goon**-dohs (mee-**noo**-tohs).

Did he / she / you lose consciousness?

¿Perdió el conocimiento?
Pehr-dee-**oh** ehl koh-noh-see-mee-**ehn**-toh?

For how long?

¿Por cuánto tiempo?
Pohr **kwahn**-toh tee-**ehm**-poh?

(X) seconds (minutes, hours).

(X) segundos (minutos, horas).
(X) seh-**goon**-dohs (mee-**noo**-tohs, oh-rahs).

Did he / she / you bite the tongue?

¿Se mordió la lengua?
Seh mohr-dee-**oh** lah **lehn**-gwah?

Was there loss of bladder or bowel control?

¿Perdió el control de la orina o excremento?
Pehr-dee-**oh** ehl kohn-**trohl** deh lah oh-**ree**-nah oh eks-kreh-**mehn**-toh?

How many attacks has he / she (have you) had today?

¿Cuántos ataques ha tenido hoy?
Kwahn-tohs ah-**tah**-kehs ah teh-**nee**-doh **oh**-ee?

Do you know if there was movement of all the extremities?

¿Sabe si hubo movimiento de todas las extremidades?
Sah-beh see **oo**-boh moh-bee-mee-**ehn**-toh deh **toh**-dahs lahs eks-treh-mee-**dah**-dehs?

Do you know if there was only movement of one side of the body?

¿Sabe si hubo movimiento de una sola parte del cuerpo?
Sah-beh see **oo**-boh moh-bee-mee-**ehn**-toh deh **oo**-nah **soh**-lah **pahr**-teh dehl **kwehr**-poh?

Was he / she (Were you) disoriented after the seizure?

¿Estaba desorientado / -a después del ataque epiléptico?
Ehs-**tah**-bah dehs-oh-ree-ehn-**tah**-doh / -dah dehs-**pwehs** dehl ah-**tah**-keh eh-pee-**lep**-tee-koh?

For how long?

¿Por cuánto tiempo?
Pohr **kwahn**-toh tee-**ehm**-poh?

(X) seconds (minutes, hours).

(X) segundos (minutos, horas).
(X) seh-**goon**-dohs (mee-**noo**-tohs, **oh**-rahs).

Do you know if there was frothing from the mouth during the seizure?

¿Sabe si había espuma en la boca durante el ataque epiléptico?
Sah-beh see ah-**bee**-ah ehs-**poo**-mah ehn lah **boh**-kah doo-**rahn**-teh ehl ah-**tah**-keh eh-pee-**lep**-tee-koh?

What was he / she (were you) doing before the attack?

¿Qué estaba haciendo antes del ataque?
Keh ehs-**tah**-bah ah-see-**ehn**-doh **ahn**-tehs dehl ah-**tah**-keh?

Drinking alcohol?

¿Estaba tomando una
bebida alcohólica?
Ehs-**tah**-bah toh-**mahn**-
doh **oo**-nah beh-**bee**-dah
ahl-**koh**-lee-kah?

Using drugs (cocaine)?

¿Estaba usando drogas
(cocaína)?
Ehs-**tah**-bah oo-**sahn**-doh
droh-gahs (koh-kah-**ee**-
nah)?

Standing?

¿Estaba parado / -a?
Ehs-**tah**-bah pah-**rah**-
doh / -dah?

Sitting?

¿Estaba sentado / -a?
Ehs-**tah**-bah sehn-**tah**-
doh / -dah?

Does he / she (Do you) have
a history of epilepsy?

¿Tiene una historia de
epilepsia?
Tee-**eh**-neh **oo**-nah ees-**toh**-
ree-ah deh eh-pee-**lep**-see-ah?

What medication does
he / she (do you) take?

¿Qué medicamento toma?
Keh meh-dee-kah-**mehn**-
toh **toh**-mah?

Dilantin?

¿Dilantin?
Dee-**lahn**-teen?

Phenobarbital?

¿Fenobarbital?
Fenoh-**bahr**-bee-tahl?

Tegretol?

¿Tégretol?
Teh-greh-tohl?

Has he / she (Have you) been
taking the seizure medication?

¿Se ha estado tomando la
medicina para los ataques?
Seh ah ehs-**tah**-doh toh-**mahn**-
doh lah me-dee-**see**-nah **pah**-
rah lohs ah-**tah**-kehs?

Before today, when was the last time he / she / you had an attack?	Antes de hoy, ¿cuándo fue la última vez que tuvo un ataque? **Ahn**-tehs deh **oh**-ee, **kwahn**-doh fweh lah **ool**-tee-mah behs keh **too**-boh oon ah-**tah**-keh?
Normally, how many attacks does he / she (do you) have a month?	Normalmente, ¿cuántos ataques tiene al mes? Nohr-mahl-**mehn**-teh, **kwahn**-tohs ah-**tah**-kehs tee-**eh**-neh ahl mehs?
Is there a history of trauma to the head?	¿Hay una historia de trauma o golpe a la cabeza? **Ah**-ee **oo**-nah ees-**toh**-ree-ah deh **trah**-oo-mah oh **gohl**-peh ah lah kah-**beh**-sah?
Are there any medical problems like . . .	¿Hay algún problema médico como... **Ah**-ee ahl-**goon** proh-**bleh**-mah **meh**-dee-koh **koh**-moh...
diabetes?	diabetes? dee-ah-**beh**-tehs?
rheumatic fever?	fiebre reumática? fee-**eh**-breh reh-oo-**mah**-tee-kah?
cardiac arrhythmias?	arritmia cardíaca? ah-**reet**-mee-ah kahr-**dee**-ah-kah?
thyroid disease?	enfermedad de la tiroides? ehn-fehr-meh-**dad** deh lah tee-**roh**-ee-dehs?

kidney disease?	enfermedad de los riñones? ehn-fehr-meh-**dad** deh lohs ree-**nyohn**-ehs?
Is he / she (Are you) on dialysis?	¿Está en diálisis? Ehs-**tah** ehn dee-**ah**-lee-sees?
cancer?	cáncer? **kahn**-sehr?

Common Phrases for the Exam for Seizures

What is your name?	¿Cuál es su nombre? Kwahl ehs soo **nohm**-breh?
	or ¿Cómo se llama? **Koh**-moh seh **yah**-mah?
What is the date today?	¿Cuál es la fecha de hoy? Kwahl ehs lah **feh**-chah deh **oh**-ee?
Do you know where you are now?	¿Sabe dónde está en este momento? **Sah**-beh **dohn**-deh ehs-**tah** ehn **ehs**-teh moh-**mehn**-toh?
What is your birth date?	¿Cuál es la fecha de su nacimiento? Kwahl ehs lah **feh**-chah deh soo nah-see-mee-**ehn**-toh?
What is your phone number?	¿Cuál es su número de teléfono? Kwahl ehs soo **noo**-meh-roh deh teh-**leh**-foh-noh?
Squeeze my hand hard.	Apriete mi mano fuerte. Ah-pree-**eh**-teh mee **mah**-noh **fwehr**-teh.

Pull me toward you.	Jáleme hacia usted. **Ha**-leh-meh **ah**-see-ah oos-**tehd**.
Raise your leg.	Levante la pierna. Leh-**bahn**-teh lah pee-**ehr**-nah.
Walk a straight line.	Camine en una línea recta. Kah-**mee**-neh ehn **oo**-nah **lee**-neh-ah **rehk**-tah.
Smile.	Sonría. Sohn-**ree**-ah.
Show me your teeth.	Muéstreme los dientes. **Mwehs**-treh-meh lohs dee-**ehn**-tehs.
Close both eyes.	Cierre ambos ojos. See-**eh**-reh **ahm**-bohs **oh**-hos.
Do you feel me touching you?	¿Siente que lo / la estoy tocando? See-**ehn**-teh keh loh / lah ehs-**toy** toh-**kahn**-doh?

Discharge Instructions for Seizures

Return to the hospital (clinic) if . . .	Regrese al hospital (a la clínica) si... Reh-**greh**-seh ahl ohs-pee-**tahl** (ah lah **klee**-nee-kah) see...
he / she continues (you continue) to have seizures,	continúan los ataques epilépticos, kohn-tee-**noo**-ahn lohs ah-**tah**-kehs eh-pee-**lep**-tee-kohs,

he / she has (you have)
trouble walking or
talking,

tiene problemas al
caminar o hablar,
tee-**eh**-neh proh-**bleh**-
mahs ahl kah-mee-**nahr**
oh ah-**blahr**,

or he / she doesn't (you
don't) have any more
seizure medication.

o no tiene más medicina
para los ataques
epilépticos.
oh noh tee-**eh**-neh mahs
meh-dee-**see**-nah **pah**-rah
lohs ah-**tah**-kehs eh-pee-
lep-tee-kohs.

Orthopedics

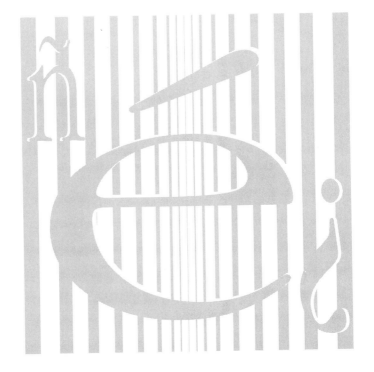

Back Pain

Dolor de Espalda

Doh-**lohr** deh ehs-**pahl**-dah

Show me where you have the pain.

Muéstreme dónde tiene el dolor.
Mwehs-treh-meh **dohn**-deh tee-**eh**-neh ehl doh-**lohr**.

Do you have pain on the right (left) side?

¿Tiene dolor en el lado derecho (izquierdo)?
Tee-**eh**-neh doh-**lohr** ehn ehl **lah**-doh deh-**reh**-choh (ees-kee-**ehr**-doh)?

Do you have pain on both sides?

¿Tiene dolor en ambos lados?
Tee-**eh**-neh doh-**lohr** ehn **ahm**-bohs **lah**-dohs?

Does the pain run to your buttock (leg)?

¿Le corre el dolor a la nalga (pierna)?
Leh **koh**-reh ehl doh-**lohr** ah lah **nahl**-gah (pee-**ehr**-nah)?

Does the pain run to your belly / groin?

¿Le corre el dolor hacia el abdomen?
Le **koh**-reh ehl doh-**lohr** ah-see-ah ehl ab-**doh**-mehn?

Does the pain run to your testicles (vagina)?

¿Le corre el dolor hacia los testículos (la vagina)?
Leh **koh**-reh ehl doh-**lohr** ah-see-ah lohs tehs-**tee**-koo-lohs (lah bah-**hee**-nah)?

When did the pain start?

¿Cuándo empezó el dolor?
Kwahn-doh ehm-peh-**soh** ehl doh-**lohr**?

How long does the pain last?	¿Cuánto tiempo le dura el dolor? **Kwahn**-toh tee-**ehm**-poh leh **doo**-rah ehl doh-**lohr**?
Have you taken medicine for the pain?	¿Ha tomado medicina para el dolor? Ah toh-**mah**-do me-dee-**see**-nah **pah**-rah ehl doh-**lohr**?
Does your leg feel asleep or numb?	¿Siente dormida o entumida la pierna? See-**ehn**-teh dohr-**mee**-dah oh ehn-too-**mee**-dah lah pee-**ehr**-nah?
Do you have weakness in the leg?	¿Tiene debilidad en la pierna? Tee-**eh**-neh deh-bee-lee-**dahd** ehn lah pee-**ehr**-nah?
Did you fall?	¿Se cayó? Seh kah-**yoh**?
When?	¿Cuándo? **Kwahn**-doh?
Today?	¿Hoy? **Oh**-ee?
Yesterday?	¿Ayer? Ah-**yehr**?
How many days (weeks) ago?	¿Hace cuántos días (cuántas semanas)? **Ah**-seh **kwahn**-tohs **dee**-ahs (**kwahn**-tahs seh-**mah**-nahs)?
Did you receive a blow to your back?	¿Recibió usted un golpe en la espalda? Reh-see-bee-**oh** oos-**tehd** oon **gohl**-peh ehn lah ehs-**pahl**-dah?

When?	¿Cuándo? **Kwahn**-doh?

Today?	¿Hoy? **Oh**-ee?

Yesterday?	¿Ayer? Ah-**yehr**?

How many days (weeks) ago?	¿Hace cuántos días (cuántas semanas)? **Ah**-seh **kwahn**-tohs **dee**-ahs (**kwahn**-tahs seh-**mah**-nahs)?

Do you have burning when you urinate?	¿Tiene ardor al orinar? Tee-**eh**-neh ahr-**dohr** ahl oh-ree-**nahr**?

Are you urinating more than normal?	¿Orina más de lo normal? Oh-**ree**-nah mahs deh loh nohr-**mahl**?

Have you noticed blood in your urine?	¿Ha notado sangre en la orina? Ah noh-**tah**-doh **sahn**-greh ehn lah oh-**ree**-nah?

Do you suffer from kidney stones?	¿Sufre usted de cálculos en los riñones? **Soo**-freh oos-**tehd** deh **kahl**-koo-lohs ehn lohs ree-**nyoh**-nehs?

Do you have problems when you urinate or have a bowel movement?	¿Tiene problemas al orinar u obrar? Tee-**eh**-neh proh-**bleh**-mahs ahl oh-ree-**nahr** oo oh-**brahr**?

Do you have pain in your abdomen?	¿Tiene dolor en el abdomen? Tee-**eh**-neh doh-**lohr** ehn ehl ab-**doh**-mehn?

Do you have a fever?	¿Tiene fiebre? Tee-**eh**-neh fee-**eh**-breh?
Do you have vomiting?	¿Tiene vómito? Tee-**eh**-neh **boh**-mee-toh?
How many times have you vomited?	¿Cuántas veces ha vomitado? **Kwahn**-tahs **beh**-sehs ah boh-mee-**tah**-doh?
How many days have you been vomiting?	¿Por cuántos días ha tenido vómito? Pohr **kwahn**-tohs **dee**-ahs ah teh-**nee**-doh **boh**-mee-toh?
Do you have pain when you cough?	¿Tiene dolor al toser? Tee-**eh**-neh doh-**lohr** ahl toh-**sehr**?
Do you have pain when you walk?	¿Tiene dolor al caminar? Tee-**eh**-neh doh-**lohr** ahl kah-mee-**nahr**?

Common Phrases for the Exam for Back Pain

Stand up and put your feet together.	Párese y ponga sus pies juntos. **Pah**-reh-seh ee **pohn**-gah soos pee-**ehs hoon**-tohs.
Touch your feet without bending your knees.	Toque sus pies sin doblar las rodillas. **Toh**-keh soos pee-**ehs** seen doh-**blahr** lahs roh-**dee**-yahs.
Move your back backwards as far as you can.	Mueva su espalda hacia atrás lo más que pueda. **Mweh**-bah soo ehs-**pahl**-dah **ah**-see-ah ah-**trahs** loh mahs keh **pweh**-dah.

Bend towards your right (left) side.	Dóblese hacia el lado derecho (izquierdo). **Doh**-bleh-seh **ah**-see-ah ehl **lah**-doh deh-**reh**-choh (ees-kee-**ehr**-doh).
Lift your right (left) leg.	Levante su pierna derecha (izquierda). Leh-**bahn**-teh soo pee-**ehr**-nah deh-**reh**-chah (ees-kee-**ehr**-dah).
We are going to get an X ray of your back.	Vamos a sacarle radiografías de la espalda. **Bah**-mohs ah sah-**kahr**-leh rah-dee-oh-grah-**fee**-ahs deh lah ehs-**pahl**-dah.
We need a urine sample.	Necesitamos una muestra de orina. Neh-seh-see-**tah**-mohs **oo**-nah **mwehs**-trah deh oh-**ree**-nah.
We are going to do a CT scan of your back.	Vamos a hacerle una tomografía (un CT) de su espalda. **Bah**-mohs ah ah-**sehr**-leh **oo**-nah toh-moh-grah-**fee**-ah (oon seh-**teh**) deh soo ehs-**pahl**-dah.
You have a kidney infection.	Usted tiene una infección del riñón. Oos-**tehd** tee-**eh**-neh **oo**-nah een-fek-see-**ohn** dehl ree-**nyohn**.
You have muscle pain.	Usted tiene dolor en los músculos. Oos-**tehd** tee-**eh**-neh doh-**lohr** ehn los **moos**-koo-lohs.

You have a fracture of a vertebra.

Usted tiene una fractura de una vértebra.

Oos-**tehd** tee-**eh**-neh **oo**-nah frak-**too**-rah deh **oo**-nah **vehr**-teh-brah.

Discharge Instructions for Back Pain

You need to rest for a day.

Usted necesita estar de reposo por un día.

Oos-**tehd** neh-seh-**see**-tah ehs-**tahr** deh reh-**poh**-soh pohr oon **dee**-ah.

Put ice on your back for 30 minutes every six hours.

Póngase hielo en la espalda por 30 minutos cada seis horas.

Pohn-gah-seh **yeh**-loh ehn lah ehs-**pahl**-dah pohr **treh**-een-tah mee-**noo**-tohs **kah**-dah **seh**-ees **oh**-rahs.

Take the medicine (X) times a day with food.

Tome la medicina (X) veces al día con comida.

Toh-meh lah meh-dee-**see**-nah (X) **beh**-sehs ahl **dee**-ah kohn koh-**mee**-dah.

Return to the hospital (clinic) if . . .

Regrese al hospital (a la clínica) si...

Reh-**greh**-seh ahl ohs-pee-**tahl** (ah lah **klee**-nee-kah) see...

you have problems urinating or moving your bowels,

tiene problemas al orinar u obrar,

tee-**eh**-neh proh-**bleh**-mahs ahl oh-ree-**nahr** oo oh-**brahr**,

you have weakness in your legs,	tiene debilidad en las piernas, tee-**eh**-neh deh-bee-lee-**dahd** ehn lahs pee-**ehr**-nahs,
you have numbness in your legs,	siente entumidas las piernas, ses-**ehn**-teh ehn-too-**mee**-dahs lahs pee-**ehr**-nahs,
you can't walk,	no puede caminar, noh **pweh**-deh kah-mee-**nahr**,
you are not better.	no se mejora. noh seh meh-**hoh**-rah.

Ankle Pain or Swelling

Dolor o Hinchazón de Tobillo

Doh-**lohr** oh een-chah-**sohn** deh toh-**bee**-yoh

Show me where the pain (swelling) is.	Enséñeme dónde tiene el dolor (la hinchazón). Ehn-**seh**-nyeh-meh **dohn**-deh tee-**eh**-neh ehl doh-**lohr** (lah een-chah-**sohn**).
When did it begin?	¿Cuándo comenzó? **Kwahn**-doh koh-mehn-**soh**?
Today.	Hoy. **Oh**-ee.
Yesterday.	Ayer. Ah-**yehr**.

(X) days (weeks) ago.	(X) días (semanas). (X) **dee**-ahs (seh-**mah**-nahs).
Did you fall?	¿Se cayó? Seh kah-**yoh**?
Did you twist your ankle?	¿Se torció el tobillo? Seh tohr-see-**oh** ehl toh-**bee**-yoh?
Did you twist it towards the inside (outside)?	¿Se lo torció hacia adentro (afuera)? Seh loh tohr-see-**oh** ah-see-ah ah-**dehn**-troh (ah-**fweh**-rah)?
Did it swell up?	¿Se le hinchó? Seh leh een-**choh**?
Did you get a bruise?	¿Se le hizo un moretón? Seh leh **ee**-soh oon moh-reh-**tohn**?
Have you taken medicine for the pain?	¿Ha tomado medicina para el dolor? Ah toh-**mah**-doh meh-dee-**see**-nah **pah**-rah ehl doh-**lohr**?
Did you put ice on the ankle?	¿Se puso hielo sobre el tobillo? Seh **poo**-soh **yeh**-loh **soh**-breh ehl toh-**bee**-yoh?
Is your ankle weak?	¿Está débil su tobillo? Ehs-**tah deh**-beel soo toh-**bee**-yoh?
Does it feel numb or asleep?	¿Lo siente entumido o dormido? Loh see-**ehn**-teh ehn-too-**mee**-doh oh dohr-**mee**-doh?

Can you walk, putting light pressure on that ankle?	¿Puede caminar, apoyando el tobillo? **Pweh**-deh kah-mee-**nahr**, ah-poh-**yahn**-doh ehl toh-**bee**-yoh?
Can you walk without pain in the ankle?	¿Puede caminar sin dolor en el tobillo? **Pweh**-deh kah-mee-**nahr** seen doh-**lohr** ehn ehl toh-**bee**-yoh?
Have you hurt the ankle before?	¿Se ha lastimado el tobillo antes? Seh ah lahs-tee-**mah**-doh ehl toh-**bee**-yoh **ahn**-tehs?

Common Phrases for the Exam for Ankle Pain or Swelling

I am going to examine your ankle.	Voy a examinarle el tobillo. **Boh**-ee ah ek-sah-mee-**nahr**-leh ehl toh-**bee**-yoh.
Does it hurt when I touch you here?	¿Le duele cuando le toco aquí? Leh **dweh**-leh **kwahn**-doh leh **toh**-koh ah-**kee**?
Move your foot . . .	Mueva su pie hacia... **Mweh**-bah soo pee-**eh ah**-see-ah...
down.	abajo. ah-**bah**-hoh.
up.	arriba. ah-**ree**-bah.
toward the inside.	adentro. ah-**dehn**-troh.

toward the outside.	afuera. ah-**fweh**-rah.
I am going to check your pulse.	Le voy a revisar el pulso. Leh **boh**-ee ah reh-bee-**sahr** ehl **pool**-soh.
You need an X ray.	Necesita una radiografía. Neh-seh-**see**-tah **oo**-nah rah-dee-oh-grah-**fee**-ah.
You need a cast.	Necesita yeso. Neh-seh-**see**-tah **yeh**-soh.
You need an Ace bandage and crutches.	Usted necesita una venda y muletas. Oos-**tehd** neh-seh-**see**-tah **oo**-nah **behn**-dah ee moo-**leh**-tahs.
You have a sprain (fracture, contusion).	Usted tiene una torcedura (fractura, contusión). Oos-**tehd** tee-**eh**-neh **oo**-nah tohr-seh-**doo**-rah (frak-**too**-rah, kohn-too-see-**ohn**).
You need surgery.	Usted necesita cirugía. Oos-**tehd** neh-seh-**see**-tah see-roo-**hee**-ah.
You need to see a bone specialist.	Usted necesita ver un especialista de los huesos. Oos-**tehd** neh-seh-**see**-tah behr oon ehs-peh-see-ah-**lees**-tah deh lohs **weh**-sohs.

Discharge Instructions for Ankle Pain or Swelling

Do not put weight on the injured foot for 48 hours.	No pise con el pie lastimado por 48 horas. Noh **pee**-seh kohn ehl pee-**eh** lahs-tee-**mah**-doh pohr koo-ah-**rehn**-tah ee **oh**-choh **oh**-rahs.

Elevate your foot as much as possible.

Eleve el pie lo más que sea posible.
Eh-**leh**-beh ehl pee-**eh** loh mahs keh **seh**-ah poh-**see**-bleh.

Put ice on your ankle for 20 minutes every six hours for two days.

Ponga hielo en el tobillo por 20 minutos cada seis horas por dos días.
Pohn-gah **yeh**-loh ehn ehl toh-**bee**-yoh pohr **beh**-een-teh mee-**noo**-tohs **kah**-dah **seh**-ees **oh**-rahs pohr dohs **dee**-ahs.

Take your medicine as indicated for the pain.

Tome la medicina como le indicaron para el dolor.
Toh-meh lah meh-dee-**see**-nah **koh**-moh leh een-dee-**kah**-rohn **pah**-rah ehl doh-**lohr**.

Return to the hospital (clinic) if . . .

Regrese al hospital (a la clínica) si...
Reh-**greh**-seh ahl ohs-pee-**tahl** (ah lah **klee**-nee-kah) see...

you have more pain,

tiene más dolor,
tee-**eh**-neh mahs doh-**lohr**,

your ankle feels numb,

el tobillo está entumido,
ehl toh-**bee**-yoh ehs-**tah** ehn-too-**mee**-doh,

your ankle is (more) swollen.

el tobillo está (más) hinchado.
ehl toh-**bee**-yoh ehs-**tah** (mahs) een-**chah**-doh.

See a specialist in (X) days (weeks).

Vaya con un especialista en (X) días (semanas).
Bah-yah kohn oon ehs-peh-see-ah-**lees**-tah ehn (X) **dee**-ahs (seh-**mah**-nahs).

Shoulder Pain or Swelling

Dolor o Hinchazón del Hombro

Doh-**lohr** oh een-chah-**sohn** dehl **ohm**-broh

Show me where the pain (swelling) is.

Enséñeme dónde tiene el dolor (la hinchazón).
Ehn-**seh**-nyeh-meh **dohn**-deh tee-**eh**-neh ehl doh-**lohr** (lah een-chah-**sohn**).

Since when have you had the pain (swelling)?

¿Desde cuándo tiene el dolor (la hinchazón)?
Dehs-deh **kwahn**-doh tee-**eh**-neh ehl doh-**lohr** (lah een-chah-**sohn**)?

For (X) days (weeks, months).

Desde (X) días (semanas, meses).
Dehs-deh (X) **dee**-ahs (seh-**mah**-nahs, **meh**-sehs).

Did you injure yourself?

¿Se lastimó?
Seh lahs-tee-**moh**?

How?

¿Cómo?
Koh-moh?

Did you fall?

¿Se cayó?
Seh kah-**yoh**?

Did you lift something heavy?

¿Levantó algo pesado?
Leh-bahn-**toh ahl**-goh peh-**sah**-doh?

Did someone hit you?

¿Alguien le pegó?
Ahl-gee-ehn leh peh-**goh**?

Were you in a car accident?	¿Estuvo en un accidente automovilístico? Ehs-**too**-boh ehn oon ak-see-**dehn**-teh ah-oo-toh-moh-bee-**lees**-tee-koh?
Were you playing sports?	¿Estaba jugando deportes? Ehs-**tah**-bah hoo-**gahn**-doh deh-**pohr**-tehs?
Did something fall on your shoulder?	¿Le cayó algo en el hombro? Leh kah-**yoh ahl**-goh en ehl **ohm**-broh?
Did it swell up?	¿Se le hinchó? Seh leh een-**choh**?
Did you get a bruise?	¿Se le hizo un moretón? Seh leh **ee**-soh oon moh-reh-**tohn**?
Have you taken medicine for the pain?	¿Ha tomado medicina para el dolor? Ah toh-**mah**-doh meh-dee-**see**-nah **pah**-rah ehl doh-**lohr**?
Did you put ice on the shoulder?	¿Se puso hielo sobre el hombro? Seh **poo**-soh **yeh**-loh **soh**-breh ehl **ohm**-broh?
Is your shoulder weak?	¿Está débil su hombro? Ehs-**tah deh**-beel soo **ohm**-broh?

Does it feel numb or asleep?	¿Lo siente entumido o dormido? Loh see-**ehn**-teh ehn-too-**mee**-doh oh dohr-**mee**-doh?
Can you lift your arm?	¿Puede levantar el brazo? **Pweh**-deh leh-bahn-**tahr** ehl **brah**-soh?
Have you hurt the shoulder before?	¿Se ha lastimado el hombro antes? Seh ah lahs-tee-**mah**-doh ehl **ohm**-broh **ahn**-tehs?
Have you dislocated the shoulder before?	¿Se ha dislocado el hombro antes? Seh ah dees-loh-**kah**-doh ehl **ohm**-broh **ahn**-tehs?

Common Phrases for the Exam for Shoulder Pain or Swelling

I am going to examine your shoulder.	Voy a examinarle el hombro. **Boh**-ee ah ek-sah-mee-**nahr**-leh ehl **ohm**-broh.
Does it hurt when I touch you here?	¿Le duele cuando le toco aquí? Leh **dweh**-leh **kwahn**-doh leh **toh**-koh ah-**kee**?
Raise your arm.	Levante el brazo. Leh-**bahn**-teh ehl **brah**-soh.
Touch the opposite shoulder with your hand.	Toque el hombro opuesto con la mano. **Toh**-keh ehl **ohm**-broh oh-**pwehs**-toh kohn lah **mah**-noh.
I am going to check your pulse.	Le voy a revisar el pulso. Leh **boh**-ee ah reh-bee-**sahr** ehl **pool**-soh.

You need an X ray.

Necesita una radiografía.
Neh-seh-**see**-tah **oo**-nah rah-
dee-oh-grah-**fee**-ah.

You have a sprain (fracture,
contusion).

Usted tiene una torcedura
(fractura, contusión).
Oos-**tehd** tee-**eh**-neh **oo**-nah
tohr-seh-**doo**-rah (frak-**too**-rah,
kohn-too-see-**ohn**).

You need surgery.

Usted necesita cirugía.
Oos-**tehd** neh-seh-**see**-tah see-
roo-**hee**-ah.

You need to see a bone
specialist.

Usted necesita ver un
especialista de los huesos.
Oos-**tehd** neh-seh-**see**-tah behr
oon ehs-peh-see-ah-**lees**-tah
deh lohs **weh**-sohs.

You dislocated your shoulder.

Se dislocó el hombro.
Seh dees-loh-**koh** ehl **ohm**-
broh.

I need to give you some
medicine to reduce the
swelling in your shoulder.

Necesito darle medicina para
reducir la hinchazón del
hombro.
Neh-seh-**see**-toh **dahr**-leh meh-
dee-**see**-nah **pah**-rah reh-doo-
seer ehl een-chah-**sohn** dehl
ohm-broh.

I need to draw some fluid
from the joint.

Necesito aspirar líquido de la
articulación.
Neh-seh-**see**-toh ahs-pee-**rahr**
lee-kee-doh deh lah ahr-tee-
koo-lah-see-**ohn**.

Discharge Instructions for Shoulder Pain or Swelling

Leave your arm in the sling.

Deje el hombro en la venda.
Deh-heh ehl **ohm**-broh ehn lah **behn**-dah.

Put ice on your shoulder for 20 minutes every six hours for two days.

Ponga hielo en el hombro por 20 minutos cada seis horas por dos días.
Pohn-gah **yeh**-loh ehn ehl **ohm**-broh pohr **beh**-een-teh mee-**noo**-tohs **kah**-dah **seh**-ees **oh**-rahs pohr dohs **dee**-ahs.

Take your medicine as indicated for the pain.

Tome la medicina como le indicaron para el dolor.
Toh-meh lah meh-dee-**see**-nah **koh**-moh leh een-dee-**kah**-rohn **pah**-rah ehl doh-**lohr**.

Return to the hospital (clinic) if . . .

Regrese al hospital (a la clínica) si...
Reh-**greh**-seh ahl ohs-pee-**tahl** (ah lah **klee**-nee-kah) see...

you have more pain,

tiene más dolor,
tee-**eh**-neh mahs doh-**lohr**,

your shoulder feels numb,

el hombro está entumido,
ehl **ohm**-broh ehs-**tah** ehn-too-**mee**-doh,

your shoulder is (more) swollen.

el hombro está (más) hinchado.
ehl **ohm**-broh ehs-**tah** (mahs) een-**chah**-doh.

See a specialist in (X) days (weeks).

Vaya con un especialista en (X) días (semanas).
Bah-yah kohn oon ehs-peh-see-ah-**lees**-tah ehn (X) **dee**-ahs (seh-**mah**-nahs).

Knee Pain or Swelling

Dolor o Hinchazón de Rodilla

Doh-**lohr** oh een-chah-**sohn** deh roh-**dee**-yah

Show me where the pain (swelling) is.

Enséñeme dónde tiene el dolor (la hinchazón).
Ehn-**seh**-nyeh-meh **dohn**-deh tee-**eh**-neh ehl doh-**lohr** (lah een-chah-**sohn**).

For how many days have you had the pain (swelling)?

¿Por cuántos días ha tenido el dolor (la hinchazón)?
Pohr **kwahn**-tohs **dee**-ahs ah teh-**nee**-doh ehl doh-**lohr** (lah een-chah-**sohn**)?

Did the pain or the swelling start first?

¿Empezó primero con el dolor o la hinchazón?
Ehm-peh-**soh** pree-**meh**-roh kohn ehl doh-**lohr** oh lah een-chah-**sohn**?

Did you injure yourself?

¿Se lastimó?
Seh lahs-tee-**moh**?

How?

¿Cómo?
Koh-moh?

Did you fall?

¿Se cayó?
Seh kah-**yoh**?

Did you twist your knee?

¿Se torció la rodilla?
Seh tohr-see-**oh** lah roh-**dee**-yah?

Did someone hit you?

¿Alguien le pegó?
Ahl-gee-ehn leh peh-**goh**?

Were you in a car accident?	¿Estuvo en un accidente automovilístico? Ehs-**too**-boh ehn oon ak-see-**dehn**-teh ah-oo-toh-moh-bee-**lees**-tee-koh?
Were you playing sports?	¿Estaba jugando deportes? Ehs-**tah**-bah hoo-**gahn**-doh deh-**pohr**-tehs?
Did your knee pop?	¿Le tronó la rodilla? Leh troh-**noh** lah roh-**dee**-yah?
Did it swell up?	¿Se le hinchó? Seh leh een-**choh**?
Have you taken medicine for the pain?	¿Ha tomado medicina para el dolor? Ah toh-**mah**-doh meh-dee-**see**-nah **pah**-rah ehl doh-**lohr**?
Did you put ice on the knee?	¿Se puso hielo sobre la rodilla? Seh **poo**-soh **yeh**-loh **soh**-breh lah roh-**dee**-yah?
Can you walk?	¿Puede caminar? **Pweh**-deh kah-mee-**nahr**?
Can you straighten out your leg?	¿Puede enderezar la pierna? **Pweh**-deh ehn-deh-reh-**sahr** lah pee-**ehr**-nah?
Does your knee feel hot?	¿Siente calor en la rodilla? See-**ehn**-teh kah-**lohr** ehn lah roh-**dee**-yah?
Do you have a fever?	¿Tiene fiebre? Tee-**eh**-neh fee-**eh**-breh?

Is your knee red or purple?	¿Tiene la rodilla roja o morada? Tee-**eh**-neh lah roh-**dee**-yah **roh**-hah oh moh-**rah**-dah?
Does it feel numb or asleep?	¿La siente entumida o dormida? Lah see-**ehn**-teh ehn-too-**mee**-dah oh dohr-**mee**-dah?
Do you have weakness in your leg?	¿Tiene debilidad en la pierna? Tee-**eh**-neh deh-bee-lee-**dahd** ehn lah pee-**ehr**-nah?
Do you have pain behind the knee?	¿Tiene dolor detrás de la rodilla? Tee-**eh**-neh doh-**lohr** deh-**trahs** deh lah roh-**dee**-yah?
Is it swollen behind the knee?	¿Tiene hinchado detrás de la rodilla? Tee-**eh**-neh een-**chah**-doh deh-**trahs** deh lah roh-**dee**-yah?
Have you hurt the knee before?	¿Se ha lastimado la rodilla antes? Seh ah lahs-tee-**mah**-doh lah roh-**dee**-yah **ahn**-tehs?
Have you had . . .	¿Ha tenido... Ah teh-**nee**-doh...
penile discharge?	deshecho del pene? dehs-**eh**-choh dehl **peh**-neh?
a venereal disease?	una enfermedad venérea? **oo**-nah ehn-fehr-meh-**dahd** beh-**neh**-reh-ah?
arthritis?	artritis? ahr-**tree**-tees?

gout?	la gota? la **goh**-tah?

Common Phrases for the Exam for Knee Pain or Swelling

I am going to examine your knee.	Voy a examinarle la rodilla. **Boh**-ee ah ek-sah-mee-**nahr**-leh lah roh-**dee**-yah.
Does it hurt when I touch you here?	¿Le duele cuando le toco aquí? Leh **dweh**-leh **kwahn**-doh leh **toh**-koh ah-**kee**?
Bend (Straighten) your knee as much as possible.	Doble (Enderece) la rodilla lo más posible. **Doh**-bleh (Ehn-deh-**reh**-seh) lah roh-**dee**-yah loh mahs poh-**see**-bleh.
I am going to check your pulse.	Le voy a revisar el pulso. Leh **boh**-ee ah reh-bee-**sahr** ehl **pool**-soh.
You need an X ray.	Necesita una radiografía. Neh-seh-**see**-tah **oo**-nah rah-dee-oh-grah-**fee**-ah.
You need a cast.	Necesita yeso. Neh-seh-**see**-tah **yeh**-soh.
You need an Ace bandage and crutches.	Usted necesita una venda y muletas. Oos-**tehd** neh-seh-**see**-tah **oo**-nah **behn**-dah ee moo-**leh**-tahs.
You have a sprain (fracture, contusion).	Usted tiene una torcedura (fractura, contusión). Oos-**tehd** tee-**eh**-neh **oo**-nah tohr-seh-**doo**-rah (frak-**too**-rah, kohn-too-see-**ohn**).

You need surgery.

Usted necesita cirugía.
Oos-**tehd** neh-seh-**see**-tah see-roo-**hee**-ah.

You need to see a bone specialist.

Usted necesita ver un especialista de los huesos.
Oos-**tehd** neh-seh-**see**-tah behr oon ehs-peh-see-ah-**lees**-tah deh lohs **weh**-sohs.

I need to draw some fluid from your knee.

Necesito aspirar líquido de su rodilla.
Neh-seh-**see**-toh ahs-pee-**rahr lee**-kee-doh deh soo roh-**dee**-yah.

You need arthroscopy.

Usted necesita artróscopia.
Oos-**tehd** neh-seh-**see**-tah ahr-**trohs**-koh-pee-ah.

You have arthritis.

Usted tiene artritis.
Oos-**tehd** tee-**eh**-neh ahr-**tree**-tees.

You have gout.

Usted tiene la gota.
Oos-**tehd** tee-**eh**-neh lah **goh**-tah.

Discharge Instructions for Knee Pain or Swelling

Do not put weight on the injured knee for 48 hours.

No pise con la rodilla lastimada por 48 horas.
Noh **pee**-seh kohn lah roh-**dee**-yah lahs-tee-**mah**-dah pohr koo-ah-**rehn**-tah ee **oh**-choh **oh**-rahs.

Elevate your knee as much as possible.

Eleve la rodilla lo más que sea posible.
Eh-**leh**-beh lah roh-**dee**-yah loh mahs keh **seh**-ah poh-**see**-bleh.

Put ice on your knee for 20 minutes every six hours for two days.

Ponga hielo en la rodilla por 20 minutos cada seis horas por dos días.
Pohn-gah **yeh**-loh ehn lah roh-**dee**-yah pohr **beh**-een-teh mee-**noo**-tohs **kah**-dah **seh**-ees **oh**-rahs pohr dohs **dee**-ahs.

Return to the hospital (clinic) if . . .

Regrese al hospital (a la clínica) si...
Reh-**greh**-seh ahl ohs-pee-**tahl** (ah lah **klee**-nee-kah) see...

you have more pain,

tiene más dolor,
tee-**eh**-neh mahs doh-**lohr**,

your knee or leg feels numb,

la rodilla o la pierna está entumida,
lah roh-**dee**-yah oh lah pee-**ehr**-nah ehs-**tah** ehn-too-**mee**-dah,

your knee is (more) swollen.

la rodilla está (más) hinchada.
la roh-**dee**-yah ehs-**tah** (mahs) een-**chah**-dah.

Elbow Pain or Swelling

Dolor o Hinchazón de Codo

Doh-**lohr** oh een-chah-**sohn** deh **koh**-doh

Show me where the pain (swelling) is.

Enséñeme dónde tiene el dolor (la hinchazón).
Ehn-**seh**-nyeh-meh **dohn**-deh tee-**eh**-neh ehl doh-**lohr** (lah een-chah-**sohn**).

For how many days have you had the pain (swelling)?

¿Por cuántos días ha tenido el dolor (la hinchazón)?

Pohr **kwahn**-tohs **dee**-ahs ah teh-**nee**-doh ehl doh-**lohr** (lah een-chah-**sohn**)?

Did the pain or the swelling start first?

¿Empezó primero con el dolor o la hinchazón?

Ehm-peh-**soh** pree-**meh**-roh kohn ehl doh-**lohr** oh lah een-chah-**sohn**?

Did you injure yourself?

¿Se lastimó?
Seh lahs-tee-**moh**?

How?

¿Cómo?
Koh-moh?

Did you fall?

¿Se cayó?
Seh kah-**yoh**?

Did you twist your elbow?

¿Se torció el codo?
Seh tohr-see-**oh** ehl **koh**-doh?

Did someone hit you?

¿Alguien le pegó?
Ahl-gee-ehn leh peh-**goh**?

Were you in a car accident?

¿Estuvo en un accidente automovilístico?
Ehs-**too**-boh ehn oon ak-see-**dehn**-teh ah-oo-toh-moh-bee-**lees**-tee-koh?

Were you playing sports?

¿Estaba jugando deportes?
Ehs-**tah**-bah hoo-**gahn**-doh deh-**pohr**-tehs?

Did something fall on your elbow?	¿Le cayó algo en el codo? Leh kah-**yoh ahl**-goh ehn ehl **koh**-doh?
Did your elbow swell up?	¿Se le hinchó el codo? Seh leh een-**choh** ehl **koh**-doh?
Have you taken medicine for the pain?	¿Ha tomado medicina para el dolor? Ah toh-**mah**-doh meh-dee-**see**-nah **pah**-rah ehl doh-**lohr**?
Did you put ice on the elbow?	¿Se puso hielo sobre el codo? Seh **poo**-soh **yeh**-loh **soh**-breh ehl **koh**-doh?
Did your elbow pop?	¿Le tronó el codo? Leh troh-**noh** ehl **koh**-doh?
Can you straighten out your elbow?	¿Puede enderezar el codo? **Pweh**-deh ehn-deh-reh-**sahr** ehl **koh**-doh?
Does your elbow feel hot?	¿Siente calor en el codo? See-**ehn**-teh kah-**lohr** ehn ehl **koh**-doh?
Do you have a fever?	¿Tiene fiebre? Tee-**eh**-neh fee-**eh**-breh?
Is your elbow red or purple?	¿Tiene el codo rojo o morado? Tee-**eh**-neh ehl **koh**-doh **roh**-hoh oh moh-**rah**-doh?
Does it feel numb or asleep?	¿Lo siente entumido o dormido? Loh see-**ehn**-teh ehn-too-**mee**-doh oh dohr-**mee**-doh?

Have you hurt the elbow before?	¿Se ha lastimado el codo antes? Seh ah lahs-tee-**mah**-doh ehl **koh**-doh **ahn**-tehs?
Have you had . . .	¿Ha tenido... Ah teh-**nee**-doh...
penile discharge?	deshecho del pene? dehs-**eh**-choh dehl **peh**-neh?
a venereal disease?	una enfermedad venérea? **oo**-nah ehn-fehr-meh-**dahd** beh-**neh**-reh-ah?
arthritis?	artritis? ahr-**tree**-tees?
gout?	la gota? lah **goh**-tah?

Common Phrases for the Exam for Elbow Pain or Swelling

I am going to examine your elbow.	Voy a examinarle el codo. **Boh**-ee ah ek-sah-mee-**nahr**-leh ehl **koh**-doh.
Does it hurt when I touch you here?	¿Le duele cuando le toco aquí? Leh **dweh**-leh **kwahn**-doh leh **toh**-koh ah-**kee**?
Bend (Straighten) your arm as much as possible.	Doble (Enderece) el brazo lo más posible. **Doh**-bleh (Ehn-deh-**reh**-seh) ehl **brah**-soh loh mahs poh-**see**-bleh.

Move your arm toward the inside (outside).	Mueva el brazo hacia adentro (afuera). **Mweh**-bah ehl **brah**-soh **ah**-see-ah ah-**dehn**-troh (ah-foo-**eh**-rah).
I am going to check your pulse.	Le voy a revisar el pulso. Leh **boh**-ee ah reh-bee-**sahr** ehl **pool**-soh.
You need an X ray.	Necesita una radiografía. Neh-seh-**see**-tah **oo**-nah rah-dee-oh-grah-**fee**-ah.
You need a cast.	Necesita yeso. Neh-seh-**see**-tah **yeh**-soh.
You need an Ace bandage.	Usted necesita una venda. Oos-**tehd** neh-seh-**see**-tah **oo**-nah **behn**-dah.
You have a sprain (fracture, contusion).	Usted tiene una torcedura (fractura, contusión). Oos-**tehd** tee-**eh**-neh **oo**-nah tohr-seh-**doo**-rah (frak-**too**-rah, kohn-too-see-**ohn**).
You need surgery.	Usted necesita cirugía. Oos-**tehd** neh-seh-**see**-tah see-roo-**hee**-ah.
You need to see a bone specialist.	Usted necesita ver un especialista de los huesos. Oos-**tehd** neh-seh-**see**-tah behr oon ehs-peh-see-ah-**lees**-tah deh lohs **weh**-sohs.
I need to draw some fluid from your elbow.	Necesito aspirar líquido de su codo. Neh-seh-**see**-toh ahs-pee-**rahr** **lee**-kee-doh deh soo **koh**-doh.

You have arthritis.

Usted tiene artritis.
Oos-**tehd** tee-**eh**-neh ahr-**tree**-tees.

You have gout.

Usted tiene la gota.
Oos-**tehd** tee-**eh**-neh lah **goh**-tah.

Discharge Instructions for Elbow Pain or Swelling

Leave your arm in the sling.

Deje su brazo en la venda.
Deh-heh soo **brah**-soh ehn lah **behn**-dah.

Elevate your arm as much as possible.

Eleve el brazo lo más que sea posible.
Eh-**leh**-beh ehl **brah**-soh loh mahs keh **seh**-ah poh-**see**-bleh.

Put ice on your elbow for 20 minutes every six hours for two days.

Ponga hielo en el codo por 20 minutos cada seis horas por dos días.
Pohn-gah **yeh**-loh ehn ehl **koh**-doh pohr **beh**-een-teh mee-**noo**-tohs **kah**-dah **seh**-ees oh-rahs pohr dohs **dee**-ahs.

Return to the hospital (clinic) if . . .

Regrese al hospital (a la clínica) si...
Reh-**greh**-seh ahl ohs-pee-**tahl** (ah lah **klee**-nee-kah) see...

you have more pain,

tiene más dolor,
tee-**eh**-neh mahs doh-**lohr**,

your elbow feels numb,

el codo está entumido,
ehl **koh**-doh ehs-**tah** ehn-too-**mee**-doh,

or your elbow is (more)
swollen.

o el codo está (más)
hinchado.
oh ehl **koh**-doh ehs-**tah**
(mahs) een-**chah**-doh.

Hand Pain or Swelling

Dolor o Hinchazón de Mano

Doh-**lohr** oh een-chah-**sohn**
deh **mah**-noh

Show me where the pain
(swelling) is.

Enséñeme dónde tiene el
dolor (la hinchazón).
Ehn-**seh**-nyeh-meh **dohn**-deh
tee-**eh**-neh ehl doh-**lohr** (lah
een-chah-**sohn**).

For how many days have you
had the pain (swelling)?

¿Por cuántos días ha tenido el
dolor (la hinchazón)?
Pohr **kwahn**-tohs **dee**-ahs ah
teh-**nee**-doh ehl doh-**lohr** (lah
een-chah-**sohn**)?

Did the pain or the swelling
start first?

¿Empezó primero con el dolor
o la hinchazón?
Ehm-peh-**soh** pree-**meh**-roh
kohn ehl doh-**lohr** oh lah een-
chah-**sohn**?

Did you injure yourself?

¿Se lastimó?
Seh lahs-tee-**moh**?

How?

¿Cómo?
Koh-moh?

Did you fall?

¿Se cayó?
Seh kah-**yoh**?

Did you twist your hand?	¿Se torció la mano? Seh tohr-see-**oh** lah **mah**-noh?
Did someone hit you?	¿Alguien le pegó? **Ahl**-gee-ehn leh peh-**goh**?
Were you in a car accident?	¿Estuvo en un accidente automovilístico? Ehs-**too**-boh ehn oon ak-see-**dehn**-teh ah-oo-toh-moh-bee-**lees**-tee-koh?
Were you playing sports?	¿Estaba jugando deportes? Ehs-**tah**-bah hoo-**gahn**-doh deh-**pohr**-tehs?
Did something fall on your hand?	¿Le cayó algo en la mano? Leh kah-**yoh ahl**-goh ehn lah **mah**-noh?
Did it swell up?	¿Se le hinchó? Seh leh een-**choh**?
Is your hand red or purple?	¿Tiene la mano roja o morada? Tee-**eh**-neh lah **mah**-noh **roh**-hah oh moh-**rah**-dah?
Have you taken medicine for the pain?	¿Ha tomado medicina para el dolor? Ah toh-**mah**-doh meh-dee-**see**-nah **pah**-rah ehl doh-**lohr**?
Did you put ice on the hand?	¿Se puso hielo sobre la mano? Seh **poo**-soh **yeh**-loh **soh**-breh lah **mah**-noh?

Does it feel numb or asleep?	¿La siente entumida o dormida? Lah see-**ehn**-teh ehn-too-**mee**-dah oh dohr-**mee**-dah?
Can you grab things with your hand?	¿Puede agarrar cosas con la mano? **Pweh**-deh ah-gah-**rar koh**-sahs kohn lah **mah**-noh?
Can you make a fist?	¿Puede hacer un puño? **Pweh**-deh ah-**sehr** oon poo-nyoh?
Have you hurt the hand before?	¿Se ha lastimado la mano antes? Seh ah lahs-tee-**mah**-doh lah **mah**-noh **ahn**-tehs?
Have you had . . .	¿Ha tenido... Ah teh-**nee**-doh...
penile discharge?	deshecho del pene? dehs-**eh**-choh dehl **peh**-neh?
a venereal disease?	una enfermedad venérea? **oo**-nah ehn-fehr-meh-**dahd** beh-**neh**-reh-ah?
arthritis?	artritis? ahr-**tree**-tees?
gout?	la gota? la **goh**-tah?

Common Phrases for the Exam for Hand Pain or Swelling

I am going to examine your hand.	Voy a examinarle la mano. **Boh**-ee ah ek-sah-mee-**nahr**-leh lah **mah**-noh.
Does it hurt when I touch you here?	¿Le duele cuando le toco aquí? Leh **dweh**-leh **kwahn**-doh leh **toh**-koh ah-**kee**?
Move your hand . . .	Mueva su mano hacia... **Mweh**-bah soo **mah**-noh **ah**-see-ah...
down.	abajo. ah-**bah**-hoh.
up.	arriba. ah-**ree**-bah.
toward the inside.	adentro. ah-**dehn**-troh.
toward the outside.	afuera. ah-**fweh**-rah.
Spread your fingers.	Separe los dedos. Seh-**pah**-reh lohs **deh**-dohs.
Put your fingers together.	Junte los dedos. **Hoon**-teh lohs **deh**-dohs.
Touch your little finger with your thumb.	Toque su dedo pequeño / meñique con el pulgar. **Toh**-keh soo **deh**-doh peh-**keh**-nyoh / meh-**nyee**-keh kohn ehl pool-**gahr**.
I am going to check your pulse.	Le voy a revisar el pulso. Leh **boh**-ee ah reh-bee-**sahr** ehl **pool**-soh.

You need an X ray.

Necesita una radiografía.
Neh-seh-**see**-tah **oo**-nah rah-dee-oh-grah-**fee**-ah.

You need a cast.

Necesita yeso.
Neh-seh-**see**-tah **yeh**-soh.

You need an Ace bandage.

Usted necesita una venda.
Oos-**tehd** neh-seh-**see**-tah **oo**-nah **behn**-dah.

You have a sprain (fracture, contusion).

Usted tiene una torcedura (fractura, contusión).
Oos-**tehd** tee-**eh**-neh **oo**-nah tohr-seh-**doo**-rah (frak-**too**-rah, kohn-too-see-**ohn**).

You need surgery.

Usted necesita cirugía.
Oos-**tehd** neh-seh-**see**-tah see-roo-**hee**-ah.

You need to see a bone specialist.

Usted necesita ver un especialista de los huesos.
Oos-**tehd** neh-seh-**see**-tah behr oon ehs-peh-see-ah-**lees**-tah deh lohs **weh**-sohs.

I need to draw some fluid from your hand.

Necesito aspirar líquido de su mano.
Neh-seh-**see**-toh ahs-pee-**rahr** **lee**-kee-doh deh soo **mah**-noh.

You have arthritis.

Usted tiene artritis.
Oos-**tehd** tee-**eh**-neh ahr-**tree**-tees.

You have gout.

Usted tiene la gota.
Oos-**tehd** tee-**eh**-neh lah **goh**-tah.

Discharge Instructions for Hand Pain or Swelling

Elevate your hand as much as possible.

Eleve la mano lo más que sea posible.
Eh-**leh**-beh lah **mah**-noh loh mahs keh **seh**-ah poh-**see**-bleh.

Put ice on your hand for 20 minutes every six hours for two days.

Ponga hielo en la mano por 20 minutos cada seis horas por dos días.
Pohn-gah **yeh**-loh ehn lah **mah**-noh pohr **beh**-een-teh mee-**noo**-tohs **kah**-dah **seh**-ees **oh**-rahs pohr dohs **dee**-ahs.

Return to the hospital (clinic) if . . .

Regrese al hospital (a la clínica) si...
Reh-**greh**-seh ahl ohs-pee-**tahl** (ah lah **klee**-nee-kah) see...

you have more pain,

tiene más dolor,
tee-**eh**-neh mahs doh-**lohr**,

your hand feels numb,

la mano está entumida,
lah **mah**-noh ehs-**tah** ehn-too-**mee**-dah,

your hand is (more) swollen.

la mano está (más) hinchada.
lah **mah**-noh ehs-**tah** (mahs) een-**chah**-dah.

Wrist Pain or Swelling

Dolor o Hinchazón de Muñeca

Doh-**lohr** oh een-chah-**sohn** deh moo-**nyeh**-kah

Show me where the pain (swelling) is.	Enséñeme dónde tiene el dolor (la hinchazón). Ehn-**seh**-nyeh-meh **dohn**-deh tee-**eh**-neh ehl doh-**lohr** (lah een-chah-**sohn**).

For how many days have you had the pain (swelling)?

¿Por cuántos días ha tenido el dolor (la hinchazón)?
Pohr **kwahn**-tohs **dee**-ahs ah teh-**nee**-doh ehl doh-**lohr** (lah een-chah-**sohn**)?

Did the pain or the swelling start first?

¿Empezó primero con el dolor o la hinchazón?
Ehm-peh-**soh** pree-**meh**-roh kohn ehl doh-**lohr** oh lah een-chah-**sohn**?

Did you injure yourself?

¿Se lastimó?
Seh lahs-tee-**moh**?

How?

¿Cómo?
Koh-moh?

Did you fall?

¿Se cayó?
Seh kah-**yoh**?

Did you twist your wrist?

¿Se torció la muñeca?
Seh tohr-see-**oh** lah moo-**nyeh**-kah?

Did someone hit you?

¿Alguien le pegó?
Ahl-gee-ehn leh peh-**goh**?

Were you in a car accident?	¿Estuvo en un accidente automovilístico? Ehs-**too**-boh ehn oon ak-see-**dehn**-teh ah-oo-toh-moh-bee-**lees**-tee-koh?
Were you playing sports?	¿Estaba jugando deportes? Ehs-**tah**-bah hoo-**gahn**-doh deh-**pohr**-tehs?
Did something fall on your wrist or hand?	¿Le cayó algo en la muñeca o en la mano? Leh kah-**yoh ahl**-goh ehn lah moo-**nyeh**-kah oh ehn lah **mah**-noh?
Did your wrist swell up?	¿Se le hinchó la muñeca? Seh leh een-**choh** lah moo-**nyeh**-kah?
Is your wrist red or purple?	¿Tiene la muñeca roja o morada? Tee-**eh**-neh lah moo-**nyeh**-kah **roh**-hah oh moh-**rah**-dah?
Have you taken medicine for the pain?	¿Ha tomado medicina para el dolor? Ah toh-**mah**-doh meh-dee-**see**-nah **pah**-rah ehl doh-**lohr**?
Did you put ice on the wrist?	¿Se puso hielo sobre la muñeca? Seh **poo**-soh **yeh**-loh **soh**-breh lah moo-**nyeh**-kah?

Does it feel numb or asleep?	¿La siente entumida o dormida? Lah see-**ehn**-teh ehn-too-**mee**-dah oh dohr-**mee**-dah?
Do you have numbness in your hand or fingers?	¿Tiene entumida la mano o los dedos? Tee-**eh**-neh ehn-too-**mee**-dah lah **mah**-noh oh lohs **deh**-dohs?
Have you hurt the wrist before?	¿Se ha lastimado la muñeca antes? Seh ah lahs-tee-**mah**-doh lah moo-**nyeh**-kah **ahn**-tehs?
Have you had . . .	¿Ha tenido... Ah teh-**nee**-doh...
penile discharge?	deshecho del pene? dehs-**eh**-choh dehl **peh**-neh?
a venereal disease?	una enfermedad venérea? **oo**-nah ehn-fehr-meh-**dahd** beh-**neh**-reh-ah?
arthritis?	artritis? ahr-**tree**-tees?
gout?	la gota? lah **goh**-tah?

Common Phrases for the Exam for Wrist Pain or Swelling

I am going to examine your wrist.	Voy a examinarle la muñeca. **Boh**-ee ah ek-sah-mee-**nahr**-leh lah moo-**nyeh**-kah.

Does it hurt when I touch you here?	¿Le duele cuando le toco aquí? Leh **dweh**-leh **kwahn**-doh leh **toh**-koh ah-**kee**?
Move your wrist . . .	Mueva su muñeca hacia... **Mweh**-bah soo moo-**nyeh**-kah **ah**-see-ah...
down.	abajo. ah-**bah**-hoh.
up.	arriba. ah-**ree**-bah.
toward the inside.	adentro. ah-**dehn**-troh.
toward the outside.	afuera. ah-**fweh**-rah.
I am going to check your pulse.	Le voy a revisar el pulso. Leh **boh**-ee ah reh-bee-**sahr** ehl **pool**-soh.
You need an X ray.	Necesita una radiografía. Neh-seh-**see**-tah **oo**-nah rah-dee-oh-grah-**fee**-ah.
You need a cast.	Necesita yeso. Neh-seh-**see**-tah **yeh**-soh.
You need an Ace bandage.	Usted necesita una venda. Oos-**tehd** neh-seh-**see**-tah **oo**-nah **behn**-dah.
You have a sprain (fracture, contusion).	Usted tiene una torcedura (fractura, contusión). Oos-**tehd** tee-**eh**-neh **oo**-nah tohr-seh-**doo**-rah (frak-**too**-rah, kohn-too-see-**ohn**).

You need surgery.

Usted necesita cirugía.
Oos-**tehd** neh-seh-**see**-tah see-roo-**hee**-ah.

You need to see a bone specialist.

Usted necesita ver un especialista de los huesos.
Oos-**tehd** neh-seh-**see**-tah behr oon ehs-peh-see-ah-**lees**-tah deh lohs **weh**-sohs.

I need to draw some fluid from your wrist.

Necesito aspirar líquido de su muñeca.
Neh-seh-**see**-toh ahs-pee-**rahr lee**-kee-doh deh soo moo-**nyeh**-kah.

You have arthritis.

Usted tiene artritis.
Oos-**tehd** tee-**eh**-neh ahr-**tree**-tees.

You have gout.

Usted tiene la gota.
Oos-**tehd** tee-**eh**-neh lah **goh**-tah.

Discharge Instructions for Wrist Pain or Swelling

Elevate your wrist as much as possible.

Eleve la muñeca lo más que sea posible.
Eh-**leh**-beh lah moo-**nyeh**-kah loh mahs keh **seh**-ah poh-**see**-bleh.

Put ice on your hand for 20 minutes every six hours for two days.

Ponga hielo en la muñeca por 20 minutos cada seis horas por dos días.
Pohn-gah **yeh**-loh ehn lah moo-**nyeh**-kah pohr **beh**-een-teh mee-**noo**-tohs **kah**-dah **seh**-ees **oh**-rahs pohr dohs **dee**-ahs.

Return to the hospital (clinic) if . . .	Regrese al hospital (a la clínica) si... **Reh-greh**-seh ahl ohs-pee-**tahl** (ah lah **klee**-nee-kah) see...
you have more pain,	tiene más dolor, tee-**eh**-neh mahs doh-**lohr**,
your hand or wrist is numb,	la mano o la muñeca está entumida, lah **mah**-noh oh lah moo-**nyeh**-kah ehs-**tah** ehn-too-**mee**-dah,
your wrist is (more) swollen.	la muñeca está (más) hinchada. lah moo-**nyeh**-kah ehs-**tah** (mahs) een-**chah**-dah.

Leg and / or Thigh Pain or Swelling

Dolor o Hinchazón de Pierna y / o Muslo

Doh-**lohr** oh een-chah-**sohn** deh **pee-ehr**-nah oh **moos**-loh

Show me where the pain (swelling) is.	Enséñeme dónde tiene el dolor (la hinchazón). Ehn-**seh**-nyeh-meh **dohn**-deh tee-**eh**-neh ehl doh-**lohr** (lah een-chah-**sohn**).
For how many days have you had the pain (swelling)?	¿Por cuántos días ha tenido el dolor (la hinchazón)? Pohr **kwahn**-tohs **dee**-ahs ah teh-**nee**-doh ehl doh-**lohr** (lah een-chah-**sohn**)?

Did the pain or the swelling start first?	¿Empezó primero con el dolor o la hinchazón? Ehm-peh-**soh** pree-**meh**-roh kohn ehl doh-**lohr** oh lah een-chah-**sohn**?
Did you injure yourself?	¿Se lastimó? Seh lahs-tee-**moh**?
How?	¿Cómo? **Koh**-moh?
Did you fall?	¿Se cayó? Seh kah-**yoh**?
Did you twist your leg?	¿Se torció la pierna? Seh tohr-see-**oh** lah pee-**ehr**-nah?
Did someone hit you?	¿Alguien le pegó? **Ahl**-gee-ehn leh peh-**goh**?
Were you in a car accident?	¿Estuvo en un accidente automovilístico? Ehs-**too**-boh ehn oon ak-see-**dehn**-teh ah-oo-toh-moh-bee-**lees**-tee-koh?
Were you playing sports?	¿Estaba jugando deportes? Ehs-**tah**-bah hoo-**gahn**-doh deh-**pohr**-tehs?
Did something fall on your leg or thigh?	¿Le cayó algo en la pierna o en el muslo? Leh kah-**yoh** ahl-goh ehn lah pee-**ehr**-nah oh ehn ehl **moos**-loh?

Did it swell up?	¿Se le hinchó? Seh leh een-**choh**?
Do you have swelling of your knee (calf)?	¿Tiene hinchada la pierna (pantorrilla)? Tee-**eh**-neh een-**chah**-dah lah pee-**ehr**-nah (pahn-toh-**ree**-yah)?
Is your leg red or purple?	¿Tiene la pierna roja o morada? Tee-**eh**-neh lah pee-**ehr**-nah **roh**-hah oh moh-**rah**-dah?
Is your thigh red or purple?	¿Tiene el muslo rojo o morado? Tee-**eh**-neh ehl **moos**-loh **roh**-hoh oh moh-**rah**-doh?
Have you taken medicine for the pain?	¿Ha tomado medicina para el dolor? Ah toh-**mah**-doh meh-dee-**see**-nah **pah**-rah ehl doh-**lohr**?
Did you put ice on the leg (thigh)?	¿Se puso hielo sobre la pierna (el muslo)? Seh **poo**-soh **yeh**-loh **soh**-breh lah pee-**ehr**-nah (ehl **moos**-loh)?
Do you have numbness in your leg or thigh?	¿Tiene entumida la pierna o el muslo? Tee-**eh**-neh ehn-too-**mee**-dah lah pee-**ehr**-nah oh ehl **moos**-loh?
Can you put weight on the leg?	¿Puede apoyar la pierna? **Pweh**-deh ah-poh-**yahr** lah pee-**ehr**-nah?
Can you walk?	¿Puede caminar? **Pweh**-deh kah-mee-**nahr**?

Have you hurt the leg (thigh) before?

¿Se ha lastimado la pierna (el muslo) antes?
Seh ah lahs-tee-**mah**-doh lah pee-**ehr**-nah (ehl **moos**-loh) **ahn**-tehs?

Common Phrases for the Exam for Leg and / or Thigh Pain or Swelling

I am going to examine your leg (thigh).

Voy a examinarle la pierna (el muslo).
Boh-ee ah ek-sah-mee-**nahr**-leh lah pee-**ehr**-nah (ehl **moos**-loh).

Does it hurt when I touch you here?

¿Le duele cuando le toco aquí?
Leh **dweh**-leh **kwahn**-doh leh **toh**-koh ah-**kee**?

Move your leg down (up).

Mueva la pierna hacia abajo (arriba).
Mweh-bah lah pee-**ehr**-nah ah-see-ah ah-**bah**-hoh (ah-**ree**-bah).

I am going to check your pulse.

Le voy a revisar el pulso.
Leh **boh**-ee ah reh-bee-**sahr** ehl **pool**-soh.

You need an X ray.

Necesita una radiografía.
Neh-seh-**see**-tah **oo**-nah rah-dee-oh-grah-**fee**-ah.

You need a cast.

Necesita yeso.
Neh-seh-**see**-tah **yeh**-soh.

You need an Ace bandage and crutches.

Usted necesita una venda y muletas.
Oos-**tehd** neh-seh-**see**-tah **oo**-nah **behn**-dah ee moo-**leh**-tahs.

You have a sprain (fracture, contusion).	Usted tiene una torcedura (fractura, contusión). Oos-**tehd** tee-**eh**-neh **oo**-nah tohr-seh-**doo**-rah (frak-**too**-rah, kohn-too-see-**ohn**).
You need surgery.	Usted necesita cirugía. Oos-**tehd** neh-seh-**see**-tah see-roo-**hee**-ah.
You need to see a bone specialist.	Usted necesita ver un especialista de los huesos. Oos-**tehd** neh-seh-**see**-tah behr oon ehs-peh-see-ah-**lees**-tah deh lohs **weh**-sohs.
You have arthritis.	Usted tiene artritis. Oos-**tehd** tee-**eh**-neh ahr-**tree**-tees.

Discharge Instructions for Leg and / or Thigh Pain or Swelling

Elevate your leg (thigh) as much as possible.	Eleve la pierna (el muslo) lo más que sea posible. Eh-**leh**-beh lah pee-**ehr**-nah (ehl **moos**-loh) loh mahs keh **seh**-ah poh-**see**-bleh.
Put ice on your leg (thigh) for 20 minutes every six hours for two days.	Ponga hielo en la pierna (el muslo) por 20 minutos cada seis horas por dos días. **Pohn**-gah **yeh**-loh ehn lah pee-**ehr**-nah (ehl **moos**-loh) pohr **beh**-een-teh mee-**noo**-tohs **kah**-dah **seh**-ees **oh**-rahs pohr dohs **dee**-ahs.

Return to the hospital (clinic) if . . .	Regrese al hospital (a la clínica) si... Reh-**greh**-seh ahl ohs-pee-**tahl** (ah lah **klee**-nee-kah) see...
you have more pain,	tiene más dolor, tee-**eh**-neh mahs doh-**lohr**,
your leg feels numb,	la pierna está entumida, lah pee-**ehr**-nah ehs-tah ehn-too-mee-dah,
your thigh feels numb,	el muslo está entumido, ehl **moos**-loh ehs-**tah** ehn-too-mee-doh,
or your leg is (more) swollen.	o la pierna está (más) hinchada. oh lah pee-**ehr**-nah ehs-**tah** (mahs) een-**chah**-dah.
your thigh is (more) swollen.	el muslo está (más) hinchado. ehl **moos**-loh ehs-**tah** (mahs) een-**chah**-doh.

Hip Pain

Dolor de Cadera

Doh-**lohr** deh kah-**deh**-rah

Show me where the pain is.	Enséñeme dónde tiene el dolor. Ehn-**seh**-nyeh-meh **dohn**-deh tee-**eh**-neh ehl doh-**lohr**.
For how many days have you had the pain?	¿Por cuántos días ha tenido el dolor? Pohr **kwahn**-tohs **dee**-ahs ah teh-**nee**-doh ehl doh-**lohr**?

Did you injure yourself?	¿Se lastimó? Seh lahs-tee-**moh**?
How?	¿Cómo? **Koh**-moh?
Did you fall?	¿Se cayó? Seh kah-**yoh**?
Did you twist your leg?	¿Se torció la pierna? Seh tohr-see-**oh** lah pee-**ehr**-nah?
Did you fall from a bed (wheelchair)?	¿Se cayó de la cama (una silla de ruedas)? seh kah-**yoh** deh lah **kah**-mah (**oo**-nah **see**-yah deh **rweh**-dahs)?
Were you in a car accident?	¿Estuvo en un accidente automovilístico? Ehs-**too**-boh ehn oon ak-see-**dehn**-teh ah-oo-toh-moh-bee-**lees**-tee-koh?
Were you playing sports?	¿Estaba jugando deportes? Ehs-**tah**-bah hoo-**gahn**-doh deh-**pohr**-tehs?
Before you fell did you have . . .	Antes de caerse, ¿tuvo... **Ahn**-tehns deh kah-**ehr**-seh, **too**-boh...
chest pain?	dolor del pecho? doh-**lohr** dehl **peh**-choh?
shortness of breath?	falta de aire? **fahl**-tah deh **ah**-ee-reh?

dizziness?	mareos?
	mah-**reh**-ohs?
a fainting spell?	desmayo?
	dehs-**mah**-yoh?
Have you taken medicine for the pain?	¿Ha tomado medicina para el dolor?
	Ah toh-**mah**-doh meh-dee-**see**-nah **pah**-rah ehl doh-**lohr**?
Can you walk?	¿Puede caminar?
	Pweh-deh kah-mee-**nahr**?
Can you straighten out your leg?	¿Puede enderezar la pierna?
	Pweh-deh ehn-deh-reh-**sahr** lah pee-**ehr**-nah?
Is your leg swollen?	¿Tiene la pierna hinchada?
	Tee-**eh**-neh lah pee-**ehr**-nah een-**chah**-dah?
Do you have a fever?	¿Tiene fiebre?
	Tee-**eh**-neh fee-**eh**-breh?
Does your leg or hip feel numb or asleep?	¿Siente entumida o dormida la pierna o cadera?
	See-**ehn**-teh ehn-too-**mee**-dah oh dohr-**mee**-dah lah pee-**ehr**-nah oh kah-**deh**-rah?
Do you have weakness in your leg?	¿Tiene debilidad en la pierna?
	Tee-**eh**-neh deh-bee-lee-**dahd** ehn lah pee-**ehr**-nah?
Have you hurt the hip before?	¿Se ha lastimado la cadera antes?
	Se ah lahs-tee-**mah**-doh lah kah-**deh**-rah **ahn**-tehs?

Have you had a hip operation before?	¿Ha tenido una operación de la cadera? Ah teh-**nee**-doh **oo**-nah oh-peh-rah-see-**ohn** deh lah kah--**deh**-rah?
Have you had . . .	¿Ha tenido... Ah teh-**nee**-doh...
penile discharge?	deshecho del pene? dehs-**eh**-choh dehl **peh**-neh?
a venereal disease?	una enfermedad venérea? **oo**-nah ehn-fehr-meh-**dahd** beh-**neh**-reh-ah?
arthritis?	artritis? ahr-**tree**-tees?
gout?	la gota? lah **goh**-tah?

Common Phrases for the Exam for Hip Pain

I am going to examine your hip.	Voy a examinarle la cadera. **Boh**-ee ah ek-sah-mee-**nahr**-leh lah kah-**deh**-rah.
Does it hurt when I touch you here?	¿Le duele cuándo le toco aquí? Leh **dweh**-leh **kwahn**-doh leh **toh**-koh ah-**kee**?
Lift your leg.	Levante la pierna. Leh-**bahn**-teh lah pee-**ehr**-nah.
Do you have pain when I move your hip?	¿Tiene dolor cuándo le muevo la cadera? Tee-**eh**-neh doh-**lohr kwahn**-doh leh **mweh**-boh lah kah-**deh**-rah?

I am going to check your pulse.

Le voy a revisar el pulso.
Leh **boh**-ee ah reh-bee-**sahr** ehl **pool**-soh.

You need an X ray.

Necesita una radiografía.
Neh-seh-**see**-tah **oo**-nah rah-dee-oh-grah-**fee**-ah.

You have a sprain (fracture, contusion).

Usted tiene una torcedura (fractura, contusión).
Oos-**tehd** tee-**eh**-neh **oo**-nah tohr-seh-**doo**-rah (frak-**too**-rah, kohn-too-see-**ohn**).

You need surgery.

Usted necesita cirugía.
Oos-**tehd** neh-seh-**see**-tah see-roo-**hee**-ah.

You need to see a bone specialist.

Usted necesita ver un especialista de los huesos.
Oos-**tehd** neh-seh-**see**-tah behr oon ehs-peh-see-ah-**lees**-tah deh lohs **weh**-sohs.

You have arthritis.

Usted tiene artritis.
Oos-**tehd** tee-**eh**-neh ahr-**tree**-tees.

We need to admit you.

Necesitamos admitirlo / -la.
Neh-seh-see-**tah**-mohs ahd-mee-**teer**-loh / -lah.

Discharge Instructions for Hip Pain

Do not put weight on the injured hip for 48 hours.

No pise con la cadera lastimada por 48 horas.
Noh **pee**-seh kohn lah kah-**deh**-rah lahs-tee-**mah**-dah pohr koo-ah-**rehn**-tah ee **oo**-choh **oh**-rahs.

Put ice on your hip for 20 minutes every six hours for two days.

Ponga hielo en la cadera por 20 minutos cada seis horas por dos días.
Pohn-gah **yeh**-loh ehn lah kah-**deh**-rah pohr **beh**-een-teh mee-**noo**-tohs **kah**-dah **seh**-ees oh-rahs pohr dohs **dee**-ahs.

Return to the hospital (clinic) if . . .

Regrese al hospital (a la clínica) si...
Reh-**greh**-seh ahl ohs-pee-**tahl** (ah lah **klee**-nee-kah) see...

you have more pain,

tiene más dolor,
tee-**eh**-neh mahs doh-**lohr**,

your knee or leg feels numb,

la rodilla o pierna está entumida,
lah roh-**dee**-yah oh pee-**ehr**-nah ehs-**tah** ehn-too-**mee**-dah,

your leg is (more) swollen.

la pierna está (más) hinchada.
la pee-**ehr**-nah ehs-**tah** (mahs) een-**chah**-dah.

Calf Pain or Swelling

Dolor o Hinchazón de Pantorilla
Doh-**lohr** oh een-chah-**sohn** deh pahn-toh-**ree**-yah

Show me where the pain (swelling) is.

Enséñeme dónde tiene el dolor (la hinchazón).
Ehn-**seh**-nyeh-meh **dohn**-deh tee-**eh**-neh ehl doh-**lohr** (lah een-chah-**sohn**).

For how many days have you had the pain (swelling)?	¿Por cuántos días ha tenido el dolor (la hinchazón)? Pohr **kwahn**-tohs **dee**-ahs ah teh-**nee**-doh ehl doh-**lohr** (lah een-chah-**sohn**)?
Did you injure yourself?	¿Se lastimó? Seh lahs-tee-**moh**?
How?	¿Cómo? **Koh**-moh?
Did you fall?	¿Se cayó? Seh kah-**yoh**?
Did you hit your leg?	¿Se pegó en la pierna? Seh peh-**goh** ehn lah pee-**ehr**-nah?
Were you playing sports?	¿Estaba jugando deportes? Ehs-**tah**-bah hoo-**gahn**-doh deh-**pohr**-tehs?
Do you have swelling in your ankle?	¿Tiene hinchado el tobillo? Tee-**eh**-neh een-**chah**-doh ehl toh-**bee**-yoh?
Do you have swelling behind the knee?	¿Tiene hinchado detrás de la rodilla? Tee-**eh**-neh een-**chah**-doh deh-**trahs** deh lah roh-**dee**-yah?
Do you have pain behind your knee?	¿Tiene dolor detrás de la rodilla? Tee-**eh**-neh doh-**lohr** deh-**trahs** deh lah roh-**dee**-yah?
Do you have pain when you walk?	¿Tiene dolor cuándo camina? Tee-**eh**-neh doh-**lohr** **kwahn**-doh kah-**mee**-nah?

Have you taken medicine for the pain?	¿Ha tomado medicina para el dolor?
	Ah toh-**mah**-doh meh-dee-**see**-nah **pah**-rah ehl doh-**lohr**?
Is your calf swollen?	¿Tiene la pantorrilla hinchada?
	Tee-**eh**-neh lah pahn-toh-**ree**-yah een-**chah**-dah?
Do you feel warmth in your calf?	¿Tiene calor en la pantorrilla?
	Tee-**eh**-neh kah-**lohr** ehn lah pahn-toh-**ree**-yah?
Do you have a fever?	¿Tiene fiebre?
	Tee-**eh**-neh fee-**eh**-breh?
Does your calf feel numb or asleep?	¿Siente entumida o dormida la pantorrilla?
	See-**ehn**-teh ehn-too-**mee**-dah oh dohr-**mee**-dah lah pahn-toh-**ree**-yah?
Do you have weakness in your leg?	¿Tiene debilidad en la pierna?
	Tee-**eh**-neh deh-bee-lee-**dahd** ehn lah pee-**ehr**-nah?
Have you hurt the calf before?	¿Se ha lastimado la pantorrilla antes?
	Seh ah lahs-tee-**mah**-doh lah pahn-toh-**ree**-yah **ahn**-tehs?
Have you recently had a long trip . . .	¿Recientemente ha hecho un viaje largo...
	Reh-see-ehn-teh-**mehn**-teh ah **eh**-choh oon bee-**ah**-heh **lahr**-goh...
in a car?	en un carro?
	ehn oon **kah**-roh?
in an airplane?	por avión?
	pohr ah-bee-**ohn**?

in a train?	por tren? pohr trehn?
Did you have an operation recently?	¿Tuvo una operación recientemente? **Too**-boh **oo**-nah oh-peh-rah-see-**ohn** reh-see-ehn-teh-**mehn**-teh?
Have you given birth recently?	¿Ha dado a luz recientemente? Ah **dah**-doh ah loos reh-see-ehn-teh-**mehn**-teh?
Have you been bedridden for a long time?	¿Ha estado encamado / -a por mucho tiempo? Ah ehs-**tah**-doh ehn-kah-**mah**-doh / -dah pohr **moo**-choh tee-**ehm**-poh?
Do you stand for a long time at work?	¿Está de pie por mucho tiempo en su trabajo? Ehs-**tah** deh pee-**eh** pohr **moo**-cho tee-**ehm**-poh ehn soo trah-**bah**-hoh?
Have you had blood clots in the leg?	¿Ha tenido coágulos de sangre en la pierna? Ah teh-**nee**-doh koh-**ah**-goo-lohs deh **sahn**-greh ehn lah pee-**ehr**-nah?
Do you have varicose veins?	¿Tiene venas varicosas? Tee-**eh**-neh **beh**-nahs bah-ree-**koh**-sahs?
Do you have problems with blood coagulation?	¿Tiene problemas con la coagulación de la sangre? Tee-**eh**-neh proh-**bleh**-mahs kohn lah koh-ah-goo-lah-see-**ohn** deh lah **sahn**-greh?
Do you smoke?	¿Fuma usted? **Foo**-mah oos-**tehd**?

Do you take birth control pills?	¿Toma anticonceptivos? ¿**Toh**-mah ahn-tee-kohn-sehp-**tee**-bohs?
Do you take Coumadin?	¿Toma usted Coumadina? **Toh**-mah oos-**tehd** koo-mah-**dee**-nah?

Common Phrases for the Exam for Calf Pain or Swelling

I am going to examine your calf.	Voy a examinarle la pantorrilla. **Boh**-ee ah ek-sah-mee-**nahr**-leh lah pahn-toh-**ree**-yah.
I am going to measure your calf.	Voy a medirle la pantorrilla. **Boh**-ee ah meh-**deer**-leh lah pahn-toh-**ree**-yah.
Does it hurt when I touch you here?	¿Le duele cuando le toco aquí? Leh **dweh**-leh **kwahn**-doh leh **toh**-koh ah-**kee**?
Do you feel pain when I move your foot?	¿Siente dolor cuando le muevo el pie? See-**ehn**-teh doh-**lohr kwahn**-doh leh **mweh**-boh ehl pee-**eh**?
Do you have pain when I touch you behind the knee?	¿Tiene dolor cuando le toco detrás de la rodilla? Tee-**eh**-neh doh-**lohr kwahn**-doh leh **toh**-koh deh-**trahs** deh lah **roh**-dee-yah?
You need an ultrasound of the leg.	Necesita un ultrasonido de la pierna. Neh-seh-**see**-tah oon ool-trah-soh-**nee**-doh deh lah pee-**ehr**-nah.

You need a venogram of the leg.	Necesita un venograma de la pierna. Neh-seh-**see**-tah oon beh-noh-**grah**-mah deh lah pee-**ehr**-nah.
You have arthritis.	Usted tiene artritis. Oos-**tehd** tee-**eh**-neh ahr-**tree**-tees.
You have a blood clot in your leg.	Usted tiene un coágulo de sangre en la pierna. Oos-**tehd** tee-**eh**-neh oon koh-**ah**-goo-loh deh **sahn**-greh ehn lah pee-**ehr**-nah.
You have a cyst behind your knee.	Usted tiene un quiste detrás de la rodilla. Oos-**tehd** tee-**eh**-neh oon **kees**-teh deh-**trahs** deh lah roh-**dee**-yah.
You need medicine to thin your blood.	Usted necesita medicina para adelgazarle la sangre. Oos-**tehd** neh-seh-**see**-tah meh-dee-**see**-nah **pah**-rah ah-dehl-gah-**sahr**-leh lah **sahn**-greh.
We need to admit you.	Necesitamos admitirlo / -la. Neh-seh-see-**tah**-mohs ahd-mee-**teer**-loh / -lah.

Discharge Instructions for Calf Pain or Swelling

Do not put weight on the injured calf for 48 hours.	No pise con la pantorrilla lastimada por 48 horas. Noh **pee**-seh kohn lah pahn-toh-**ree**-yah lahs-tee-**mah**-dah pohr koo-ah-**rehn**-tah ee **oh**-choh **oh**-rahs.

Put ice on your calf for 20 minutes every six hours for two days.

Ponga hielo en la pantorrilla por 20 minutos cada seis horas por dos días.
Pohn-gah **yeh**-loh ehn lah pahn-toh-**ree**-yah pohr **beh**-een-teh mee-**noo**-tohs **kah**-dah **seh**-ees **oh**-rahs pohr dohs **dee**-ahs.

Elevate your leg as much as possible.

Eleve su pierna lo más que sea posible.
Eh-**leh**-beh soo pee-**ehr**-nah loh mahs keh **seh**-ah poh-**see**-bleh.

Take your medicine as indicated.

Tome su medicina como le fue indicado.
Toh-meh soo meh-dee-**see**-nah **koh**-moh leh fweh een-dee-**kah**-doh.

See your doctor in (X) days.

Consulte con su médico en (X) días.
Kohn-**sool**-teh kohn soo **meh**-dee-koh ehn (X) **dee**-ahs.

Return to the hospital (clinic) if . . .

Regrese al hospital (a la clínica) si...
Reh-**greh**-seh ahl ohs-pee-**tahl** (ah lah **klee**-nee-kah) see...

you have more pain,

tiene más dolor,
tee-**eh**-neh mahs doh-**lohr**,

your calf or leg feels numb,

la pantorrilla o pierna está entumida,
lah pahn-toh-**ree**-yah oh pee-**ehr**-nah ehs-**tah** ehn-too-**mee**-dah,

your leg is (more) swollen,	la pierna está (más) hinchada, la pee-**ehr**-nah ehs-**tah** (mahs) een-**chah**-dah,
your calf or leg changes color.	la pantorrilla o pierna cambia de color. lah pahn-toh-**ree**-yah oh pee-**ehr**-nah **kahm**-bee-ah deh koh-**lohr**.

Foot Pain or Swelling

Dolor o Hinchazón de Pie

Doh-**lohr** oh een-chah-**sohn** deh pee-**eh**

Show me where the pain (swelling) is.	Enséñeme dónde tiene el dolor (la hinchazón). Ehn-**seh**-nyeh-meh **dohn**-deh tee-**eh**-neh ehl doh-**lohr** (lah een-chah-**sohn**).
When did it begin?	¿Cuándo comenzó? **Kwahn**-doh koh-mehn-**soh**?
Today?	¿Hoy? **Oh**-ee?
Yesterday?	¿Ayer? Ah-**yehr**?
(X) days (weeks) ago?	¿(X) días (semanas)? (X) **dee**-ahs (seh-**mah**-nahs)?
Did you fall?	¿Se cayó? Seh kah-**yoh**?

Did you twist your foot toward the inside (outside)?	¿Se torció el pie hacia adentro (afuera)?
	Seh tohr-see-**oh** ehl pee-**eh** ah-see-ah ah-**dehn**-troh (ah-**fweh**-rah)?
Did it swell up?	¿Se le hinchó?
	Seh leh een-**choh**?
Did you get a bruise?	¿Se le hizo un moretón?
	Seh leh **ee**-soh oon moh-reh-**tohn**?
Have you taken medicine for the pain?	¿Ha tomado medicina para el dolor?
	Ah toh-**mah**-doh meh-dee-**see**-nah **pah**-rah ehl doh-**lohr**?
Did you put ice on the foot?	¿Se puso hielo sobre el pie?
	Seh **poo**-soh **yeh**-loh **soh**-breh ehl pee-**eh**?
Is your foot weak?	¿Esta débil su pie?
	Ehs-tah **deh**-beel soo peeh-**eh**?
Does it feel numb or asleep?	¿Lo siente entumido o dormido?
	Loh see-**ehn**-teh ehn-too-**mee**-doh oh dohr-**mee**-doh?
Can you walk, putting light pressure on that foot?	¿Puede caminar apoyando el pie?
	Pweh-deh kah-mee-**nahr** ah-poh-**yahn**-doh ehl pee-**eh**?
Can you walk without pain in the foot?	¿Puede caminar sin dolor en el pie?
	Pweh-deh kah-mee-**nahr** seen doh-**lohr** ehn ehl pee-**eh**?
Have you hurt the foot before?	¿Se ha lastimado el pie antes?
	Seh ah lahs-tee-**mah**-doh ehl pee-**eh** ahn-tehs?

Common Phrases for the Exam for Foot Pain or Swelling

I am going to examine your foot.	Voy a examinarle el pie. **Boh**-ee ah ek-sah-mee-**nahr**-leh ehl pee-**eh**.
Does it hurt when I touch you here?	¿Le duele cuando le toco aquí? Leh **dweh**-leh **kwahn**-doh leh **toh**-koh ah-**kee**?
Move your foot . . .	Mueva su pie hacia... **Mweh**-bah soo pee-**eh ah**-see-ah...
down.	abajo. ah-**bah**-hoh.
up.	arriba. ah-**ree**-bah.
toward the inside.	adentro. ah-**dehn**-troh.
toward the outside.	afuera. ah-**fweh**-rah.
I am going to check your pulse.	Le voy a revisar el pulso. Leh **boh**-ee ah reh-bee-**sahr** ehl **pool**-soh.
You need an X ray.	Necesita una radiografía. Neh-seh-**see**-tah **oo**-nah rah-dee-oh-grah-**fee**-ah.
You need a cast.	Necesita yeso. Neh-seh-**see**-tah **yeh**-soh.

You have a sprain (fracture, contusion).	Usted tiene una torcedura (fractura, contusión). Oos-**tehd** tee-**eh**-neh **oo**-nah tohr-seh-**doo**-rah (frak-**too**-rah, kohn-too-see-**ohn**).
You need surgery.	Usted necesita cirugía. Oos-**tehd** neh-seh-**see**-tah see-roo-**hee**-ah.
You need to see a bone specialist.	Usted necesita ver un especialista de los huesos. Oos-**tehd** neh-seh-**see**-tah behr oon ehs-peh-see-ah-**lees**-tah deh lohs **weh**-sohs.
You need an Ace bandage and crutches.	Usted necesita una venda y muletas. Oos-**tehd** neh-seh-**see**-tah **oo**-nah **behn**-dah ee moo-**leh**-tahs.

Discharge Instructions for Foot Pain or Swelling

Do not put weight on the injured foot for 48 hours.	No pise con el pie lastimado por 48 horas. Noh **pee**-seh kohn ehl pee-**eh** lahs-tee-**mah**-doh pohr koo-ah-**rehn**-tah ee **oh**-choh **oh**-rahs.
Elevate your foot as much as possible.	Eleve el pie lo más que sea posible. Eh-**leh**-beh ehl pee-**eh** loh mahs keh **seh**-ah poh-**see**-bleh.
Put ice on your foot for 20 minutes every six hours for two days.	Ponga hielo en el pie por 20 minutos cada seis horas por dos días. **Pohn**-gah **yeh**-loh ehn ehl pee-**eh** pohr **beh**-een-teh mee-**noo**-tohs **kah**-dah **seh**-ees **oh**-rahs pohr dohs **dee**-ahs.

Take your medicine as indicated for the pain.	Tome la medicina como le indicaron para el dolor. **Toh**-meh lah meh-dee-**see**-nah **koh**-moh leh een-dee-**kah**-rohn **pah**-rah ehl doh-**lohr**.
Return to the hospital (clinic) if . . .	Regrese al hospital (a la clínica) si... Reh-**greh**-seh ahl ohs-pee-**tahl** (ah lah **klee**-nee-kah) see...
you have more pain,	tiene más dolor, tee-**eh**-neh mahs doh-**lohr**,
your foot feels numb,	el pie está entumido, ehl pee-**eh** ehs-**tah** ehn-too-**mee**-doh,
your foot is (more) swollen.	el pie está (más) hinchado. ehl pee-**eh** ehs-**tah** (mahs) een-**chah**-doh.
See a specialist in (X) days (weeks).	Vaya con un especialista en (X) días (semanas). **Bah**-yah kohn oon ehs-peh-see-ah-**lees**-tah ehn (X) **dee**-ahs (seh-**mah**-nahs).

Miscellaneous

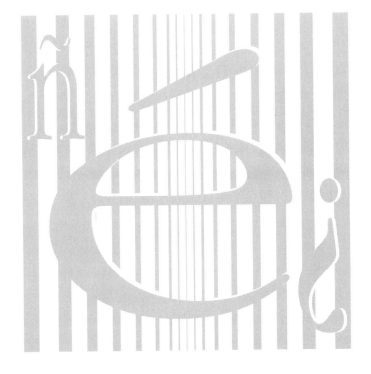

Diabetic Patient

El Paciente con Diabetes

Ehl pah-see-**ehn**-teh kohn dee-ah-**beh**-tehs

Do you know if you have diabetes?

¿Usted sabe si tiene diabetes?
Oos-**tehd sah**-beh see tee-**eh**-neh dee-ah-**beh**-tehs?

Are you urinating more than normal?

¿Orina más de lo normal?
Oh-**ree**-nah mahs deh loh nohr-**mahl**?

Are you more thirsty than normal?

¿Tiene más sed de lo normal?
Tee-**eh**-neh mahs sehd deh loh nohr-**mahl**?

Have you lost weight in the past weeks?

¿Ha perdido peso en las últimas semanas?
Ah pehr-**dee**-doh **peh**-soh ehn lahs **ool**-tee-mahs seh-**mah**-nahs?

Have you gained weight in the last weeks?

¿Ha aumentado de peso en las últimas semanas?
Ah ah-oo-mehn-**tah**-doh deh **peh**-soh ehn lahs **ool**-tee-mahs seh-**mah**-nahs?

Are you more hungry than normal?

¿Tiene más hambre de lo normal?
Tee-**eh**-neh mahs **ahm**-breh deh loh nohr-**mahl**?

Do you take insulin (diabetic pills)?

¿Toma insulina (píldoras para la diabetes)?
Toh-mah een-soo-**lee**-nah (**peel**-doh-rahs **pah**-rah lah dee-ah-**beh**-tehs)?

What type of insulin do you take?	¿Qué tipo de insulina toma?
	Keh **tee**-poh deh een-soo-**lee**-nah **toh**-mah?
Regular?	¿Regular?
	Reh-goo-**lahr**?
NPH?	¿NPH?
	Eh-neh Peh **Ah**-cheh?
Humulin 70 / 30?	¿Humulina 70 / 30?
	Oo-moo-**lee**-nah seh-**tehn**-tah **treh**-een-tah?
How many units of insulin do you take in the morning (evening)?	¿Cuántas unidades de insulina toma en la mañana (tarde)?
	Kwahn-tahs oo-nee-**dah**-dehs deh een-soo-**lee**-nah **toh**-mah ehn lah mah-**nyah**-nah (**tahr**-deh)?
When was the last time you took your medicine?	¿Cuándo fue la última vez que tomó su medicina?
	Kwahn-doh fweh lah **ool**-tee-mah behs keh toh-**moh** soo meh-dee-**see**-nah?
At (X) o'clock.	A las (X).
	Ah lahs (X).
This morning.	Esta mañana.
	Ehs-tah mah-**nyah**-nah.
Last night.	Anoche.
	Ah-**noh**-cheh.

(X) hours (days, weeks) ago.	(X) horas (días, semanas). (X) **oh**-rahs (**dee**-ahs, seh-**mah**-nahs).
Have you eaten breakfast?	¿Ha desayunado? Ah dehs-ah-yoo-**nah**-doh?
Have you eaten lunch?	¿Ha almorzado (merendado, tomado el lonche)? Ah ahl-mohr-**sah**-doh (meh-rehn-**dah**-doh, toh-**mah**-doh ehl **lohn**-cheh)?
Have you eaten dinner / supper?	¿Ha cenado (tomado la comida)? Ah seh-**nah**-doh (toh-**mah**-doh lah koh-**mee**-dah)?
Do you have abdominal pain?	¿Tiene dolor abdominal? Tee-**eh**-neh doh-**lohr** ab-doh-mee-**nahl**?
Do you have nausea or vomiting?	¿Tiene náusea o vómito? Tee-**eh**-neh **nah**-oo-seh-ah oh **boh**-mee-toh?
Do you have chest pain?	¿Tiene dolor del pecho? Tee-**eh**-neh doh-**lohr** dehl **peh**-choh?
Do you feel dizzy?	¿Se siente mareado / -a? Seh see-**ehn**-teh mah-reh-**ah**-doh / -dah?
Do you check your blood sugar level at home?	¿Usted revisa en casa el nivel de azúcar de la sangre? Oos-**tehd** reh-**bee**-sah ehn **kah**-sah ehl nee-**behl** deh ah-**soo**-kahr deh lah **sahn**-greh?

| What was the blood sugar when you checked it? | ¿Cuánto fue el azúcar cuándo lo revisó?
Kwahn-toh fweh ehl ah-**soo**-kahr **kwan**-doh loh reh-bee-**soh**? |

Common Phrases for the Exam for Diabetes

You have diabetes.	Usted tiene diabetes. Oos-**tehd** tee-**eh**-neh dee-ah-**beh**-tehs.
Your blood sugar level is very high.	Usted tiene muy alto el nivel de azúcar de la sangre. Oos-**tehd** tee-**eh**-neh **moo**-ee **ahl**-toh ehl nee-**behl** deh ah-**soo**-kahr deh lah **sahn**-greh.
You need to take insulin.	Usted necesita tomar insulina. Oos-**tehd** neh-seh-**see**-tah toh-**mahr** een-soo-**lee**-nah.
You need intravenous fluids.	Usted necesita líquidos intravenosos. Oos-**tehd** neh-seh-**see**-tah **lee**-kee-dohs een-trah-beh-**noh**-sohs.
You need a fasting blood sugar test tomorrow (in two days, next week).	Necesita hacer una prueba de azúcar de la sangre en ayunas mañana (en dos días, la semana que viene). Neh-seh-**see**-tah ah-**sehr** oo-nah **prweh**-bah deh ah-**soo**-kahr deh lah **sahn**-greh ehn ah-**yoo**-nahs mah-**nyah**-nah (ehn dohs **dee**-ahs, lah seh-**mah**-nah keh bee-**en**-neh).

Discharge Instructions for the Diabetic Patient

Take your medicine.

Tome su medicina.
Toh-meh soo meh-dee-**see**-nah.

Avoid sweet foods.

Evite las comidas dulces.
Eh-**bee**-teh lahs koh-**mee**-dahs **dool**-sehs.

Return to the hospital (clinic) if . . .

Regrese al hospital (a la clínica) si...
Reh-**greh**-seh ahl ohs-pee-**tahl** (ah lah **klee**-nee-kah) see...

you have vomiting,

tiene vómito,
tee-**eh**-neh **boh**-mee-toh,

you are dizzy,

está mareado / -a,
ehs-**tah** mah-reh-**ah**-doh / -dah,

your blood sugar level is very high.

el nivel de azúcar de la sangre está muy alto.
ehl nee-**behl** deh ah-**soo**-kahr deh lah **sahn**-greh ehs-**tah moo**-ee ahl-toh.

Motor Vehicle Accident (Crash)

Accidente Automovilístico (Choque)

Ak-see-**dehn**-teh oo-toh-moh-bee-**lees**-tee-koh (**choh**-keh)

When did the accident occur?

¿Cuándo ocurrió el accidente?
Kwahn-doh oh-koo-ree-**oh** ehl ak-see-**dehn**-teh?

(X) hours (days, weeks) ago.	(X) horas (días, semanas). (X) **oh**-rahs (**dee**-ahs, seh-**mah**-nahs).
Were you the passenger?	¿Usted fue el pasajero (la pasajera)? Oos-**tehd** fweh ehl pah-sah-**heh**-roh (lah pah-sah-**heh**-rah)?
Were you the driver?	¿Usted fue el conductor (la conductora)? Oos-**tehd** fweh ehl kohn-dook-**tohr** (lah kohn-dook-**toh**-rah)?
Where in the car were you sitting?	¿Dónde estaba sentado / -a? **Dohn**-deh ehs-**tah**-bah sehn-**tah**-doh / -dah?
In front?	¿Enfrente? Ehn-**frehn**-teh?
In back?	¿Atrás? Ah-**trahs**?
Were you wearing your seat belt?	¿Tenía puesto su cinturón de seguridad? Teh-**nee**-ah **pwehs**-toh soo seen-too-**rohn** deh seh-goo-ree-**dad**?
At what speed was your car going?	¿A qué velocidad iba su coche / auto? Ah keh beh-lo-see-**dahd ee**-bah soo **koh**-cheh / **ah**-oo-toh?
Was the crash head on?	¿El choque fue de frente? Ehl **choh**-keh fweh deh **frehn**-teh?
Was the crash from behind?	¿El choque fue por detrás? Ehl **choh**-keh fweh pohr deh-**trahs**?

Was the crash from the driver's (passenger's) side?	¿El choque fue por el lado del conductor (pasajero)?
	Ehl **choh**-keh fweh pohr ehl **lah**-doh dehl kohn-dook-**tohr** (pah-sah-**heh**-roh)?
Was the crash on the street or highway?	¿El choque fue en la calle o autopista?
	Ehl **choh**-keh fweh ehn lah **kah**-yeh o ah-oo-toh-**pees**-tah?
Was anyone killed in the accident?	¿Se mató alguien en el accidente?
	Seh mah-**toh ahl**-gee-ehn ehn ehl ak-see-**dehn**-teh?
Did you hit the windshield?	¿Se pegó usted contra el parabrisas?
	Seh peh-**goh** oos-**tehd kohn**-trah ehl pah-rah-**bree**-sahs?
Did you crack the windshield?	¿Rajó / Estrelló el parabrisas?
	Rah-**hoh** / Ehs-treh-**yoh** ehl pah-rah-**bree**-sahs?
Did you hit your chest against the steering wheel?	¿Se pegó el pecho contra el volante?
	Seh peh-**goh** ehl **peh**-choh **kohn**-trah ehl boh-**lahn**-teh?
Did you get cut?	¿Se cortó?
	Seh kohr-**toh**?
Show me where.	¿Enséñeme dónde.
	Ehn-**seh**-nyeh-meh **dohn**-deh.

When was the last time you received a tetanus vaccine?

¿Cuándo fue la última vez que recibió una vacuna del tétano?
Kwahn-doh fweh lah **ool**-tee-mah behs keh reh-see-bee-**oh oo**-nah bah-**koo**-nah dehl **teh**-tah-noh?

(X) months (years) ago.

(X) meses (años).
(X) **meh**-sehs (**ah**-nyohs).

When I was young (a child).

Cuando era joven (niño / a).
Koo-**ahn**-doh **eh**-rah **hoh**-behn (**nee**-nyoh / -nyah).

I don't know (remember).

No sé (recuerdo).
Noh seh (reh-koo-**ehr**-doh).

Did you lose consciousness?

¿Perdió el conocimiento?
Pehr-dee-**oh** ehl koh-noh-see-mee-**ehn**-toh?

For how long did you lose consciousness?

¿Por cuánto tiempo perdió el conocimiento?
Pohr **kwahn**-toh tee-**ehm**-poh pehr-dee-**oh** ehl koh-noh-see-mee-**ehn**-toh?

For (X) seconds (minutes, hours).

Por (X) segundos (minutos, horas).
Pohr (X) seh-**goon**-dohs (mee-**noo**-tohs, **oh**-rahs).

Do you have neck pain?

¿Tiene dolor en el cuello?
Tee-**eh**-neh doh-**lohr** ehn ehl **kweh**-yoh?

Do you have numbness or tingling in your hands (legs)?

¿Tiene dormidas / entumidas u hormigueo en las manos (piernas)?
Tee-**eh**-neh dohr-**mee**-dahs / ehn-too-**mee**-dahs oo ohr-mee-**geh**-oh ehn lahs **mah**-nohs (pee-**ehr**-nahs)?

Do you have numbness or tingling in your arms?

¿Tiene dormidos / entumidos o hormigueo en los brazos?
Tee-**eh**-neh dohr-**mee**-dohs / ehn-too-**mee**-dohs oh ohr-mee-**geh**-oh ehn lohs **brah**-sohs?

Do you have a headache?

¿Tiene dolor de cabeza?
Tee-**eh**-neh doh-**lohr** deh kah-**beh**-sah?

Have you vomited since the accident?

¿Ha vomitado desde el accidente?
Ah boh-mee-**tah**-doh **dehs**-deh ehl ak-see-**dehn**-teh?

Do you have blurred vision?

¿Tiene la vista nublada o borrosa?
Tee-**eh**-neh lah **bees**-tah noo-**blah**-dah oh boh-**roh**-sah?

Does your side (back, chest) hurt?

¿Le duele el costado (la espalda, el pecho)?
Leh **dweh**-leh ehl koh-**stah**-doh (lah ehs-**pahl**-dah, ehl **peh**-choh)?

Do your ribs hurt?

¿Le duelen las costillas?
Leh **dweh**-lehn lahs kohs-**tee**-yahs?

Do you feel short of breath?

¿Siente que le falta la respiración?
See-**ehn**-teh keh leh **fahl**-tah lah rehs-pee-rah-see-**ohn**?

Do you hurt anywhere else?	¿Tiene dolor en cualquier otro lugar? Tee-**eh**-neh doh-**lohr** ehn kwahl-kee-**ehr oh**-troh loo-**gahr**?
Have you noticed blood in your urine?	¿Ha notado sangre en la orina? Ah noh-**tah**-doh **sahn**-greh ehn lah oh-**ree**-nah?
Do you have any medical problems such as . . .	¿Tiene algún problema médico como... Tee-**eh**-neh ahl-**goon** proh-**bleh**-mah **meh**-dee-koh **koh**-moh...
high blood pressure?	alta presión de la sangre? **ahl**-tah preh-see-**ohn** deh lah sahn-greh?
diabetes?	diabetes? dee-ah-**beh**-tehs?
heart disease?	alguna enfermedad del corazón? ahl-**goo**-nah ehn-fehr-meh-**dahd** dehl koh-rah-**sohn**?
epilepsy?	epilepsia? eh-pee-**lep**-see-ah?
asthma?	asma? **ahs**-mah?
Do you take any medicine?	¿Toma alguna medicina? **Toh**-mah ahl-**goo**-nah meh-dee-**see**-nah?
Do you have any allergies?	¿Tiene alguna alergia? Tee-**eh**-neh ahl-**goo**-nah ah-**lehr**-hee-ah?

Are you allergic to penicillin (aspirin, ibuprofen)?	Es alérgico / -a a la penicilina (la aspirina, el ibuprofen)? **Ehs** ah-**lehr**-hee-koh / -kah ah lah peh-nee-see-**lee**-nah (lah ahs-pee-**ree**-nah, ehl ee-boo-**proh**-fehn)?
Have you been drinking alcohol?	¿Ha estado tomando bebidas alcohólicas? Ah ehs-**tah**-doh toh-**mahn**-doh beh-**bee**-dahs ahl-**koh**-lee-kahs?

Common Phrases for the Exam for Motor Vehicle Accident

Look at the light.	Mire la luz. **Mee**-reh lah loos.
Follow my finger with your eyes, without moving your head.	Siga mi dedo con los ojos, sin mover la cabeza. **See**-gah mee **deh**-doh kohn lohs **oh**-hohs, seen moh-**behr** lah kah-**beh**-sah.
Show me where you have pain.	Muéstreme dónde tiene dolor. **Mwehs**-treh-meh **dohn**-deh tee-**eh**-neh doh-**lohr**.
Don't move your head.	No mueva la cabeza. Noh **mweh**-bah lah kah-**beh**-sah.
Lift your right (left) leg.	Levante la pierna derecha (izquierda). Leh-**bahn**-teh lah pee-**ehr**-nah deh-**reh**-chah (ees-kee-**ehr**-dah).

Squeeze my hand.	Apriete mi mano. Ah-pree-**eh**-teh mee **mah**-noh.
Pull me toward you.	Jáleme hacia usted. **Ha**-leh-meh **ah**-see-ah oos-**tehd.**
Tell me if you have pain when I touch your neck.	Dígame si tiene dolor cuando le toco el cuello. **Dee**-gah-meh see tee-**eh**-neh doh-**lohr kwahn**-doh leh **toh**-koh ehl **kweh**-yoh.
Do not move your neck.	No mueva el cuello. Noh **mweh**-bah ehl **kweh**-yoh.
I am going to put a hard collar on your neck.	Le voy a poner un collar en el cuello. Leh **boh**-ee ah poh-**nehr** oon koh-**yahr** ehn ehl **kweh**-yoh.
Tell me if you have pain when I move your pelvic bone.	Dígame si tiene dolor cuando le muevo el hueso pélvico. **Dee**-gah-meh see tee-**eh**-neh doh-**lohr kwahn**-doh leh **mweh**-boh ehl **weh**-soh **pel**-bee-koh.
We are going to get an X ray of your neck.	Vamos a tomarle una radiografía del cuello. **Bah**-mohs ah toh-**mahr**-leh oo-nah rah-dee-oh-grah-**fee**-ah dehl **kweh**-yoh.
We are going to get an X ray (CT) of your head.	Vamos a tomarle una radiografía (tomografía) de la cabeza. **Bah**-mohs ah toh-**mahr**-leh oo-nah rah-dee-oh-grah-**fee**-ah (toh-moh-grah-**fee**-ah) deh lah kah-**beh**-sah.

Discharge Instructions for Motor Vehicle Accident

Take the medicine (X) times a day with food.

Tome la medicina (X) veces al día con comida.
Toh-meh lah meh-dee-**see**-nah (X) **beh**-sehs ahl **dee**-ah kohn koh-**mee**-dah.

Return to the hospital (clinic) if you have . . .

Regrese al hospital (a la clínica) si tiene...
Reh-**greh**-seh ahl ohs-pee-**tahl** (ah lah **klee**-nee-kah) see tee-**eh**-neh...

more pain,

más dolor,
mahs doh-**lohr**,

headache,

dolor de cabeza,
doh-**lohr** deh kah-**beh**-sah,

vomiting,

vómito,
boh-mee-toh,

blurred vision,

la vista borrosa,
lah **bees**-tah boh-**roh**-sah,

numbness in the arms and legs,

entumidos los brazos y piernas,
ehn-too-**mee**-dohs lohs **brah**-sohs ee pee-**ehr**-nahs,

weakness in the arms and legs.

debilidad en los brazos y piernas.
deh-bee-lee-**dahd** ehn lohs **brah**-sohs ee pee-**ehr**-nahs.

Overdose	**Sobredosis**
	Soh-breh-**doh**-sees
How many pills have you taken?	¿Cuántas pastillas ha tomado? **Kwahn**-tahs pahs-**tee**-yahs ah **toh**-mah-doh?
What pills did you take?	¿Qué pastillas tomó? Keh pahs-**tee**-yahs toh-**moh**?
Aspirin?	¿Aspirinas? Ahs-pee-**ree**-nahs?
Tylenol?	¿Tylenol? **Tay**-leh-nohl?
Ibuprofen?	¿Ibuprofen? Ee-boo-**proh**-fehn?
Antibiotics?	¿Antibióticos? Ahn-tee-bee-**oh**-tee-kohs?
Hypertension pills?	¿Pastillas para la presión? Pahs-**tee**-yahs **pah**-rah lah preh-see-**ohn**?
Antidepressants?	¿Pastillas para la depresión? Pahs-**tee**-yahs **pah**-rah lah deh-preh-see-**ohn**?
Dilantin?	¿Dilantin? Dee-**lahn**-teen?
Something else?	¿Alguna otra cosa? Ahl-**goo**-nah **oh**-trah **koh**-sah?

What time did you take the pills?	¿A qué hora tomó las pastillas? Ah keh **oh**-rah toh-**moh** lahs pahs-**tee**-yahs?
Did you bring the pill bottles with you?	¿Trajo con usted los frascos de pastillas? **Trah**-hoh kohn oos-**tehd** lohs **frahs**-kohs deh pahs-**tee**-yahs?
Did you drink alcohol?	¿Tomó bebidas alcohólicas? Toh-**moh** beh-**bee**-dahs ahl-**koh**-lee-kahs?
Did you take the pills to kill yourself?	¿Tomó las pastillas para matarse? Toh-**moh** lahs pahs-**tee**-yahs **pah**-rah mah-**tahr**-seh?
Do you still want to kill yourself?	¿Todavía quiere matarse? Toh-dah-**bee**-ah kee-**eh**-reh mah-**tahr**-seh?
Have you tried to kill yourself before?	¿Ha tratado de matarse antes? Ah trah-**tah**-doh deh mah-**tahr**-seh **ahn**-tehs?
Do you suffer from depression?	¿Sufre de depresión? **Soo**-freh deh deh-preh-see-**ohn**?
Why did you want to kill yourself?	¿Por qué quizo matarse? Pohr keh **kee**-soh mah-**tahr**-seh?
Problems at work?	¿Problemas en el trabajo? Proh-**bleh**-mahs ehn ehl trah-**bah**-hoh?
Marriage problems?	¿Problemas del matrimonio? Proh-**bleh**-mahs dehl mah-tree-**moh**-nee-oh?

Personal problems?	¿Problemas personales? Proh-**bleh**-mahs pehr-soh-**nah**-lehs?
Something else?	¿Otra cosa? Oh-trah **koh**-sah?
Have you used illegal drugs recently?	¿Ha tomado drogas ilegales recientemente? Ah toh-**mah**-doh **droh**-gahs ee-leh-gah-lehs reh-see-ehn-teh-**mehn**-teh?
Marihuana?	¿Marijuana? Mah-ree-**hwah**-nah?
Cocaine?	¿Cocaína? Koh-kah-**ee**-nah?
Heroin?	¿Heroína? Eh-roh-**ee**-nah?
A different drug?	¿Otra droga? **Oh**-trah **droh**-gah?
Do you have abdominal pain?	¿Tiene dolor abdominal? Tee-**eh**-neh doh-**lohr** ab-doh-mee-**nahl**?
Do you have nausea or vomiting?	¿Tiene náusea o vómito? Tee-**eh**-neh **nah**-oo-seh-ah oh **boh**-mee-toh?
Have you vomited since taking the pills?	¿Ha vomitado desde que tomó las pastillas? Ah boh-mee-**tah**-doh **dehs**-deh keh toh-**moh** lahs pahs-**tee**-yahs?
Are you dizzy?	¿Tiene mareos? Tee-**eh**-neh mah-**reh**-ohs?

Common Phrases for the Exam for Overdose

I need to put a tube through your mouth to empty your stomach.	Necesito ponerle un tubo por la boca para vaciarle el estómago. Neh-seh-**see**-toh poh-**nehr**-leh oon **too**-boh pohr lah **boh**-kah **pah**-rah bah-see-**ahr**-leh ehl ehs-**toh**-mah-goh.
You need a nasogastric tube.	Necesita una sonda nasogástrica. Neh-seh-**see**-tah **oo**-nah **sohn**-dah nah-soh-**gahs**-tree-kah.
You need to take medicine to neutralize the pills you took.	Necesita tomar medicina para neutralizar las pastillas que tomó. Neh-seh-**see**-tah toh-**mahr** meh-dee-**see**-nah **pah**-rah neh-oo-trah-lee-**sahr** lahs pahs-**tee**-yahs keh toh-**moh**.
You need to see a psychiatrist.	Usted necesita ver un psiquiatra. Oos-**tehd** neh-seh-**see**-tah behr oon see-kee-**ah**-trah.
We need to admit you.	Necesitamos internarlo / -la. Neh-seh-see-**tah**-mohs een-tehr-**nahr**-loh / -lah.

Discharge Instructions for Overdose

Return to the hospital (clinic) if . . .	Regrese al hospital (a la clínica) si... Reh-**greh**-seh ahl ohs-pee-**tahl** (ah lah **klee**-nee-kah) see...

you have abdominal pain, vomiting, or dizziness,

tiene dolor abdominal, vómito, o mareos,
tee-**eh**-neh doh-**lohr** ab-doh-mee-**nahl**, **boh**-mee-toh, oh mah-**reh**-ohs,

or feel like hurting yourself or others.

o siente que va a lastimarse a sí o a otros.
oh see-**ehn**-teh keh bah ah lahs-tee-**mahr**-seh ah see oh ah **oh**-trohs.

Depression or Suicidal Ideation

Depresión o Ideas Suicidas

Deh-preh-**see-ohn** oh ee-deh-ahs soo-ee-see-dahs

Are you depressed?

¿Está usted deprimido / -a?
Ehs-**tah** oos-**tehd** deh-pree-**mee**-doh / -dah?

How long have you been depressed?

¿Por cuánto tiempo ha estado deprimido / -a?
Pohr **kwahn**-toh tee-**ehm**-poh ah ehs-**tah**-doh deh-**pree**-mee-doh / -dah?

For (X) days (weeks, months, years).

Por (X) días (semanas, meses, años).
Pohr (X) **dee**-ahs (seh-**mah**-nahs, **meh**-sehs, **ah**-nyohs).

Do you have trouble sleeping?

¿Tiene dificultades para dormir?
Tee-**eh**-neh dee-fee-kool-**tah**-dehs **pah**-rah dohr-**meer**?

How many hours a day do you sleep?

¿Cuántas horas duerme al día?
Kwahn-tahs **oh**-rahs **dwehr**-meh ahl **dee**-ah?

Do you wake up at dawn?

¿Se levanta en la madrugada?
Seh leh-**bahn**-tah ehn lah mah-droo-**gah**-dah?

Is there a lack of appetite?

¿Tiene falta de apetito?
Tee-**eh**-neh **fahl**-tah deh ah-peh-**tee**-toh?

Have you lost interest in sex?

¿Ha perdido interés en el sexo?
Ah pehr-**dee**-doh een-teh-**rehs** ehn ehl **sek**-soh?

Do you cry for any reason?

¿Llora usted por cualquier cosa?
Yoh-rah oos-**tehd** pohr kwahl-kee-**ehr koh**-sah?

Do you feel without value?

¿Siente que no tiene valor?
See-**ehn**-teh keh noh tee-**eh**-neh bah-**lohr**?

Do you hear voices that no one else can hear?

¿Oye usted voces que no oyen los demás?
Oh-yeh oos-**tehd boh**-sehs keh noh **oh**-yehn lohs deh-**mahs**?

When did you start hearing voices?

¿Cuándo empezó a oír voces?
Kwahn-doh ehm-peh-**soh** ah oh-**eer boh**-sehs?

(X) days (weeks, months, years) ago.

(X) días (semanas, meses, años).
(X) **dee**-ahs (seh-**mah**-nahs, **meh**-sehs, **ah**-nyohs).

Do the voices tell you to hurt or kill yourself?

¿Le dicen las voces que se lastime o que se suicide?
Leh **dee**-sehn lahs **boh**-sehs keh seh lahs-**tee**-meh oh keh seh soo-ee-**see**-deh?

Do the voices tell you to hurt other people?

¿Le dicen las voces que lastime a otras personas?
Leh **dee**-sehn lahs **boh**-sehs keh lahs-**tee**-meh ah **oh**-trahs pehr-**soh**-nahs?

Have you ever tried to kill yourself?

¿Alguna vez ha tratado de matarse?
Ahl-**goo**-nah behs ah trah-**tah**-doh deh mah-**tahr**-seh?

When?

¿Cuándo?
Kwahn-doh?

What month?

¿En qué mes?
Ehn keh mehs?

What year?

¿En qué año?
Ehn keh **ah**-nyoh?

How many times have you tried to kill yourself?

¿Cuántas veces ha intentado matarse?
Kwahn-tahs **beh**-sehs ah een-tehn-**tah**-doh mah-**tahr**-seh?

How did you try to kill yourself?

¿Cómo trató de matarse?
Koh-moh trah-**toh** deh mah-**tahr**-seh?

With pills?

¿Con pastillas?
Kohn pahs-**tee**-yahs?

With a knife?

¿Con un cuchillo?
Kohn oon koo-**chee**-yoh?

With a gun?

¿Con una pistola o un rifle?
Kohn **oo**-nah pees-**toh**-lah oh oon **ree**-fleh?

Jumping from a high place?

¿Saltando de un lugar alto?
Sahl-**tahn**-doh deh oon loo-**gahr ahl**-toh?

By hanging yourself?

¿Ahorcándose?
Ah-ohr-**kahn**-doh-seh?

Do you still want to kill yourself?

¿Todavía quiere matarse?
Toh-dah-**bee**-ah kee-**eh**-reh mah-**tahr**-seh?

Do you think that the TV or radio is speaking only to you?

¿Cree que la televisión o la radio le habla solamente a usted?
Kreh-eh keh lah teh-leh-bee-see-**ohn** oh lah **rah**-dee-oh leh **ah**-blah soh-lah-**mehn**-teh ah oos-**tehd**?

Do you think that someone is following you?

¿Cree que alguien le persigue?
Kreh-eh keh **ahl**-gee-ehn leh pehr-**see**-geh?

Do you think that people are talking behind your back?

¿Cree que la gente habla de usted a sus espaldas?
Kreh-eh keh lah **hehn**-teh **ah**-blah deh oos-**tehd** ah soos ehs-**pahl**-dahs?

Have you been seen by a psychiatrist?	¿Lo / La ha visto un psiquiatra?
	Loh / Lah ah **bees**-toh oon see-kee-**ah**-trah?
Have you been admitted to a psychiatric hospital?	¿Lo / La han internado en un hospital psiquiátrico?
	Loh / Lah ahn een-tehr-**nah**-doh ehn oon ohs-pee-**tahl** see-kee-**ah**-tree-koh?
Are you taking medication such as . . .	¿Está tomando medicina como...
	Ehs-**tah** toh-**mahn**-doh meh-dee-**see**-nah **koh**-moh...
Haldol?	Haldol?
	Hal-dohl?
Elavil?	Elavil?
	Eh-lah-beel?
Prolixin?	Prolixin?
	Proh-**leek**-seen?
Thorazine?	Thorazine?
	Toh-rah-seen?
Valium?	Valium?
	Bah-lee-oom?
Do you drink alcohol?	¿Toma usted bebidas alcohólicas?
	Toh-mah oos-**tehd** beh-**bee**-dahs ahl-**koh**-lee-kahs?
When was the last time you drank?	¿Cuándo fue la última vez que tomó?
	Kwahn-doh fweh lah **ool**-tee-mah behs keh toh-**moh**?
Do you use drugs such as . . .	¿Usa drogas como...
	Oo-sah **droh**-gahs **koh**-moh...

marihuana?	marijuana? mah-ree-**hwah**-nah?
cocaine?	cocaína? koh-kah-**ee**-nah?
crack cocaine?	rocas de cocaína? **roh**-kahs de koh-kah-**ee**-nah?
heroin (inhaled or IV)?	heroína (inhalada o intravenosa)? eh-roh-**ee**-nah (een-ah-**lah**-dah oh een-trah-beh-**noh**-sah)?
mushrooms?	hongos? **ohn**-gohs?

Common Phrases for the Exam for Depression or Suicidal Ideation

You need to see a psychiatrist.	Usted necesita ver un psiquiatra. Oos-**tehd** neh-seh-**see**-tah behr oon see-kee-**ah**-trah.
We need to restrain you for your protection.	Necesitamos atarlo / -la para su protección. Neh-seh-see-**tah**-mohs ah-**tahr**-loh / -lah **pah**-rah soo proh-tek-see-**ohn**.
We are going to send you to a psychiatric hospital.	Vamos a mandarlo / -la a un hospital psiquiátrico. **Bah**-mohs ah mahn-**dahr**-loh / -lah ah oon ohs-pee-**tahl** see-kee-**ah**-tree-koh.

We are going to give you pills for the depression.	Vamos a darle pastillas para la depresión.
	Bah-mohs ah **dahr**-leh pahs-**tee**-yahs **pah**-rah lah deh-preh-see-**ohn**.

Discharge Instructions for Depression or Suicidal Ideation

Take the medicine as indicated.	Tome la medicina como le indicaron.
	Toh-meh lah meh-dee-**see**-nah **koh**-moh leh een-dee-**kah**-rohn.
See a psychiatrist soon.	Consulte con un psiquiatra pronto.
	Kohn-sool-teh kohn oon see-kee-**ah**-trah **prohn**-toh.
Return to the hospital (clinic) if . . .	Regrese al hospital (a la clínica) si...
	Reh-**greh**-seh al ohs-pee-**tahl** (ah lah **klee**-nee-kah) see...
you still feel depressed,	todavía se siente deprimido / -a,
	toh-dah-**bee**-ah seh see-**ehn**-teh deh-pree-**mee**-doh / -dah,
you think you are going to hurt yourself,	piensa que se va a lastimar,
	pee-**ehn**-sah keh seh bah ah lahs-tee-**mahr**,
you think you are going to hurt others.	piensa que va a lastimar a otros.
	pee-**ehn**-sah keh bah ah lahs-tee-**mahr** ah **oh**-trohs.

Animal Bite

Mordidas de Animales

Mohr-**dee**-dahs deh ah-nee-**mah**-lehs

When were you bitten?

¿Cuándo lo / la mordieron?

Kwahn-doh loh / lah mohr-dee-**eh**-rohn?

Did it turn red around the wound?

¿Se puso rojo alrededor de la herida?

Seh **poo**-soh **roh**-hoh ahl-reh-deh-**dohr** deh lah eh-**ree**-dah?

Does the wound feel numb or asleep?

¿Siente entumida o dormida la herida?

See-**ehn**-teh ehn-too-**mee**-dah oh dohr-**mee**-dah lah eh-**ree**-dah?

Does it hurt?

¿Tiene dolor?

Tee-**eh**-neh doh-**lohr**?

Does it itch?

¿Tiene comezón?

Tee-**eh**-neh koh-meh-**sohn**?

Is there pus in the wound?

¿Hay pus en la herida?

Ah-ee poos ehn lah eh-**ree**-dah?

What animal bit you?

¿Qué animal lo / la mordió?

Keh ah-nee-**mahl** loh / lah mohr-dee-**oh**?

A dog?

¿Un perro?

Oon **peh**-roh?

A cat?

¿Un gato?

Oon **gah**-toh?

A squirrel?	¿Una ardilla? **Oo**-nah ahr-**dee**-yah?
A mouse or rat?	¿Un ratón o una rata? Oon rah-**tohn** oh oo-nah **rah**-tah?
Another animal?	¿Otro animal? **Oh**-troh ah-nee-**mahl**?
Do you know the animal that bit you?	¿Conoce al animal que lo / la mordió? Koh-**noh**-seh ahl ah-nee-**mahl** keh loh / lah mohr-dee-**oh**?
Do you know if the animal is vaccinated?	¿Sabe si está vacunado el animal? **Sah**-beh see ehs-**tah** bah-koo- **nah**-doh ehl ah-nee-**mahl**?
Did you report the attack to the police?	¿Reportó el ataque a la policía? Reh-pohr-**toh** ehl ah-**tah**-keh ah lah poh-lee-**see**-ah?
When was your last tetanus shot?	¿Cuándo fue su última vacuna del tétano? **Kwahn**-doh fweh soo **ool**-tee- mah bah-**koo**-nah dehl **teh**-tah- noh?

Common Phrases for the Exam for an Animal Bite

We have to clean the wound.	Tenemos que limpiarle la herida. Teh-**neh**-mohs keh leem-pee- **ahr**-leh lah eh-**ree**-dah.

You need sutures to close the wound.

Usted necesita puntadas para cerrar la herida.

Oos-**tehd** neh-seh-**see**-tah poon-**tah**-dahs **pah**-rah seh-**rahr** lah eh-**ree**-dah.

You need a tetanus vaccine.

Usted necesita una vacuna del tétano.

Oos-**tehd** neh-seh-**see**-tah **oo**-nah bah-**koo**-nah dehl **teh**-tah-noh.

You need an antibiotic injection.

Usted necesita una injección de antibiótico.

Oos-**tehd** neh-seh-**see**-tah **oo**-nah een-yek-see-**ohn** deh ahn-tee-bee-**oh**-tee-koh.

You (do not) need a rabies vaccine.

Usted (no) necesita una vacuna para la rabia.

Oos-**tehd** (noh) neh-seh-**see**-tah **oo**-nah bah-**koo**-nah **pah**-rah lah **rah**-bee-ah.

I am not going to suture the wound so it doesn't become infected.

No voy a darle puntadas para que no se le infecte la herida.

Noh **boh**-ee ah **dahr**-leh poon-**tah**-dahs **pah**-rah keh noh seh leh een-**fek**-teh lah eh-**ree**-dah.

Discharge Instructions for an Animal Bite

Keep the wound clean and dry.

Mantenga limpia y seca la herida.

Mahn-**tehn**-gah **leem**-pee-ah ee **seh**-kah lah eh-**ree**-dah.

Return to the hospital (clinic) if . . .

Regrese al hospital (a la clínica) si...

Reh-**greh**-seh ahl ohs-pee-**tahl** (ah lah **klee**-nee-kah) see...

the wound turns red,	la herida se pone roja, lah eh-**ree**-dah seh **poh**-neh **roh**-hah,
there is pus from the wound,	hay pus de la herida, **ah**-ee poos deh lah eh-**ree**-dah,
you have a lot of pain or swelling,	hay mucho dolor o hinchazón, **ah**-ee **moo**-choh doh-**lohr** oh een-chah-**sohn**,
you have a fever,	tiene fiebre, tee-**eh**-neh fee-**eh**-breh,
an extremity becomes numb.	se pone entumida una extremidad. seh **poh**-neh een-too-**mee**-dah oo-nah eks-treh-mee-**dahd**.

Burns

Quemaduras

Keh-mah-doo-rahs

How did you burn yourself?	¿Con qué se quemó? Kohn keh seh keh-**moh**?
With hot water?	¿Con agua caliente? Kohn **ah**-gwah kah-lee-**ehn**-teh?
With hot oil?	¿Con aceite caliente? Kohn ah-**seh**-ee-teh kah-lee-**ehn**-teh?
With a house radiator?	¿Con un radiador de casa? Kohn oon rah-dee-ah-**dohr** deh **kah**-sah?

With an iron?	¿Con una plancha?
	Kohn **oo**-nah **plahn**-chah?

On the stove?	¿Con la estufa?
	Kohn lah ehs-**too**-fah?

On the car radiator?	¿Con el radiador del coche?
	Kohn ehl rah-dee-ah-**dohr** dehl koh-cheh?

With acid?	¿Con ácido?
	Kohn **ah**-see-doh?

With fire?	¿Con fuego?
	Kohn **fweh**-goh?

When did you burn yourself?	¿Cuándo se quemó?
	Kwahn-doh seh keh-**moh**?

(X) hours (days, weeks) ago.	(X) horas (días, semanas).
	(X) **oh**-rahs (**dee**-ahs, seh-**mah**-nahs).

Do you have pain?	¿Tiene dolor?
	Tee-**eh**-neh doh-**lohr**?

Does the burned area feel numb or asleep?	¿Siente entumida o dormida el area quemada?
	See-**ehn**-teh ehn-too-**mee**-dah oh dohr-**mee**-dah ehl **ah**-reh-ah keh-**mah**-dah?

Have you noticed any pus from the burn?	¿Ha notado pus en la quemadura?
	Ah noh-**tah**-doh poos ehn lah keh-mah-**doo**-rah?

Do you have a fever?	¿Tiene fiebre?
	Tee-**eh**-neh fee-**eh**-breh?

When was the last time you received a tetanus vaccine?

¿Cuándo fue la última vez que recibió una vacuna del tétano?
Kwahn-doh fweh lah **ool**-tee-mah behs keh reh-see-bee-**oh** **oo**-nah bah-**koo**-nah dehl **teh**-tah-noh?

Do you have allergies?

¿Tiene alergias?
Tee-**eh**-neh ah-**lehr**-hee-ahs?

Common Phrases for the Exam for Burns

We are going to clean your burn.

Vamos a limpiarle la quemadura.
Bah-mohs ah leem-pee-**ahr**-leh lah keh-mah-**doo**-rah.

We are going to put a special cream on the burn.

Vamos a ponerle una crema especial sobre la quemadura.
Bah-mohs ah poh-**nehr**-leh oo-nah **kreh**-mah ehs-peh-see-**ahl** **soh**-breh lah keh-mah-**doo**-rah.

Discharge Instructions for Burns

Change your dressings every day and apply Silvadine.

Cambie sus vendajes / gasas todos los días y aplique Silvadine.
Kahm-bee-eh soos behn-**dah**-hehs / **gah**-sahs **toh**-dohs lohs **dee**-ahs ee ah-**plee**-keh Seel-bah-**deen**.

Return to the hospital (clinic) if you have . . .

Regrese al hospital (a la clínica) si tiene...
Reh-**greh**-seh ahl ohs-pee-**tahl** (ah lah **klee**-nee-kah) see tee-**eh**-neh...

a fever,

fiebre,
fee-**eh**-breh,

a lot of pain,	mucho dolor, **moo**-choh doh-**lohr**,
discharge from the burn,	deshecho de la quemadura, dehs-**eh**-choh deh lah keh-mah-**doo**-rah,
redness around the burn.	rojo alrededor de la quemadura. **roh**-hoh ahl-reh-deh-**dohr** deh lah keh-mah-**doo**-rah.

Smoke Inhalation

Inhalación de Humo

Een-ah-lah-**see-ohn** deh **oo**-moh

How long were you in the smoke?	¿Cuánto tiempo estuvo en el humo? **Kwahn**-toh tee-**ehm**-poh ehs-**too**-boh ehn ehl **oo**-moh?
Was there ventilation in the room?	¿Había ventilación en el cuarto? Ah-**bee**-ah behn-tee-lah-see-**ohn** ehn ehl **kwahr**-toh?
Do you feel short of breath?	¿Siente falta de aire? See-**ehn**-teh **fahl**-tah deh **ah**-ee-reh?
Do you have a cough?	¿Tiene tos? Tee-**eh**-neh tohs?
Do you have phlegm?	¿Tiene flema? Tee-**eh**-neh **fleh**-mah?

Have you noticed black phlegm?	¿Ha notado flema negra? Ah noh-**tah**-doh **fleh**-mah **neh**-grah?
Do you have wheezing in your chest?	¿Tiene silbidos en el pecho? Tee-**eh**-neh seel-**bee**-dohs ehn ehl **peh**-choh?
Do you have pain in your throat?	¿Tiene dolor en la garganta? Tee-**eh**-neh doh-**lohr** ehn lah gahr-**gahn**-tah?
Are you hoarse?	¿Está ronco / -a? Ehs-**tah rohn**-koh / -kah?
Does your chest hurt?	¿Le duele el pecho? Leh **dweh**-leh ehl **peh**-choh?
Do you feel dizzy?	¿Se siente mareado / -a? Seh see-**ehn**-teh mah-reh-**ah**-doh / -dah?
Do you have a headache?	¿Tiene dolor de cabeza? Tee-**eh**-neh doh-**lohr** deh kah-**beh**-sah?
Does any part of your body feel numb?	¿Siente entumida alguna parte de su cuerpo? See-**ehn**-teh ehn-too-**mee**-dah ahl-**goo**-nah **pahr**-teh deh soo **kwerh**-poh?
Do you have nausea or vomiting?	¿Tiene náusea o vómito? Tee-**eh**-neh **nah**-oo-seh-ah oh **boh**-mee-toh?
(*for a woman*) When was your last period?	¿Cuándo fue su última regla? **Kwahn**-doh fweh soo **ool**-tee-mah **reh**-glah?
Are you pregnant?	¿Está embarazada? Ehs-**tah** ehm-bah-rah-**sah**-dah?

Common Phrases for the Exam for Smoke Inhalation

I need to do an arterial blood test.	Necesito hacerle una prueba de sangre arterial. Neh-seh-**see**-toh ah-**sehr**-leh **oo**-nah **prweh**-bah deh **sahn**-greh ahr-teh-ree-**ahl**.
We need to take an X ray.	Necesitamos sacarle una radiografía (unos rayos X). Neh-seh-see-**tah**-mos sah-**kahr**-leh **oo**-nah rah-dee-oh-grah-**fee**-ah (**oo**-nos **rah**-yohs **eh**-keys).
We need to intubate you.	Necesitamos intubarlo / la. Neh-seh-see-**tah**-mohs een-too-**bahr**-loh / -lah.
You need oxygen.	Usted necesita oxígeno. Oos-**tehd** neh-seh-**see**-tah ohk-**see**-heh-noh.

Discharge Instructions for Smoke Inhalation

Return to the hospital (clinic) if . . .	Regrese al hospital (a la clínica) si... Reh-**greh**-seh ahl ohs-pee-**tahl** (ah lah **klee**-nee-kah) see...
you have a headache or are dizzy,	tiene dolor de cabeza o está mareado / -a, tee-**eh**-neh doh-**lohr** deh kah-**beh**-sah oh ehs-**tah** mah-reh-**ah**-doh / -dah,
you are short of breath,	tiene falta de aire, Tee-**eh**-neh **fahl**-tah deh **ah**-ee-reh,

you feel choked,	se siente sofocado / -a, seh see-**ehn**-teh soh-foh-**kah**-doh / -dah,
you have wheezing in your chest.	tiene silbidos en el pecho. tee-**eh**-neh seel-**bee**-dohs ehn ehl **peh**-choh.

Laceration

Laceración
Lah-seh-rah-**see**-ohn

How long ago did you get cut?	¿Cuánto tiempo hace que se cortó? **Kwahn**-toh tee-**ehm**-poh **ah**-seh keh seh kohr-**toh**?
(X) minutes (hours, days, weeks) ago.	(X) minutos (horas, días, semanas). (X) mee-**noo**-tohs (**oh**-rahs, **dee**-ahs, seh-**mah**-nahs).
What did you get cut with?	¿Con qué se cortó? Kohn keh seh kohr-**toh**?
With a knife?	¿Con un cuchillo? Kohn oon koo-**chee**-yoh?
With a switch blade?	¿Con una navaja? Kohn **oo**-nah nah-**bah**-hah?
With a razor blade?	¿Con una hoja / navaja de afeitar? Kohn **oo**-nah **oh**-hah / nah-**bah**-hah deh ah-feh-ee-**tahr**?

With broken glass or a broken bottle?	¿Con vidrio roto o una botella rota? Kohn **bee**-dree-oh roh-toh oh **oo**-nah boh-**teh**-yah **roh**-tah?
With a broken mirror?	¿Con un espejo roto? Kohn oon ehs-**peh**-hoh **roh**-toh?
With wood?	¿Con madera? Kohn mah-**deh**-rah?
With metal?	¿Con metal? Kohn meh-**tahl**?
Do you have numbness in your . . .	¿Tiene entumido o adormecido... Tee-**eh**-neh ehn-too-**mee**-doh oh ah-dohr-meh-**see**-doh...
arm?	el brazo? ehl **brah**-soh?
forearm?	el antebrazo? ehl ahn-teh-**brah**-soh?
finger?	el dedo? ehl **deh**-doh?
thigh?	el muslo? ehl **moos**-lo?
foot?	el pie? ehl pee-**eh**?
Do you have numbness in your . . .	¿Tiene entumida o adormecida... Tee-**eh**-neh ehn-too-**mee**-dah oh ah-dohr-meh-**see**-dah...
face?	la cara? la **kah**-rah?

| hand? | la mano? |
| | lah **mah**-noh? |

| leg? | la pierna? |
| | lah pee-**ehr**-nah? |

| Do you have numbness in your . . . | ¿Tiene entumidos o adormecidos... |
| | Tee-**eh**-neh ehn-too-**mee**-dohs oh ah-dohr-meh-**see**-dohs... |

| fingers? | los dedos? |
| | lohs **deh**-dohs? |

| toes? | los dedos de los pies? |
| | lohs **deh**-dohs deh lohs pee-**ehs**? |

| Do you have weakness in an extremity? | ¿Tiene usted debilidad en una extremidad? |
| | Tee-**eh**-neh oos-**tehd** deh-bee-lee-**dahd** ehn **oo**-nah eks-treh-mee-**dahd**? |

| Does the wound hurt? | ¿Le duele la herida? |
| | Leh **dweh**-leh lah eh-**ree**-dah? |

| Do you feel something inside the wound? | ¿Siente algo dentro de la herida? |
| | See-**ehn**-teh **ahl**-goh **dehn**-troh deh lah eh-**ree**-dah? |

| Is there redness around the wound? | ¿Está rojo alrededor de la herida? |
| | Ehs-**tah roh**-hoh ahl-reh-deh-**dohr** deh lah eh-**ree**-dah? |

| Do you have drainage from the wound? | ¿Tiene usted deshecho de la herida? |
| | Tee-**eh**-neh oos-**tehd** dehs-**eh**-choh deh lah eh-**ree**-dah? |

What color is the drainage?	¿De qué color es el deshecho? Deh keh koh-**lohr** ehs ehl dehs-**eh**-choh?
Is it yellow?	¿Es amarillo? Ehs ah-mah-**ree**-yoh?
Is it red?	¿Es rojo? Ehs **roh**-hoh?
Is it clear?	¿Es claro? Ehs **klah**-roh?
When was the last time you received a tetanus vaccine?	¿Cuándo fue la última vez que recibió una vacuna del tétano? **Kwanh**-doh fweh lah **ool**-tee-mah behs keh reh-see-bee-**oh** **oo**-nah bah-**koo**-nah dehl **teh**-tah-noh?
Do you have any medical problems such as . . .	¿Tiene usted algún problema médico como... Tee-**eh**-neh oos-**tehd** ahl-**goon** proh-**bleh**-mah **meh**-dee-koh **koh**-moh...
diabetes?	diabetes? dee-ah-**beh**-tehs?
AIDS?	el SIDA? ehl **see**-dah?
bad circulation?	mala circulación de la sangre? **mah**-lah seer-koo-lah-see-**ohn** deh lah **sahn**-greh?
blood that doesn't clot?	sangre que no se coagula? **sahn**-greh keh noh seh koo-ah-**goo**-lah?

Do you take blood thinners?	¿Toma usted medicina para adelgazarle la sangre? **Toh**-mah oos-**tehd** meh-dee-**see**-nah **pah**-rah ah-dehl-gah-**sahr**-leh lah **sahn**-greh?
Do you take Coumadin?	¿Toma Coumadina? **Toh**-mah Koo-mah-**dee**-nah?
Do you take aspirin?	¿Toma aspirinas? **Toh**-mah ahs-pee-**ree**-nahs?
Are you allergic to any antibiotics?	¿Es usted alérgico / -a a algún antibiótico? Ehs oos-**tehd** ah-**lehr**-hee-koh / -kah ah ahl-**goon** ahn-tee-bee-**oh**-tee-koh?
Are you allergic to anesthetics?	¿Es usted alérgico / -a a algún anestésico? Ehs oos-**tehd** ah-**lehr**-hee-koh / -kah ah ahl-**goon** ah-nehs-**teh**-see-koh?

Common Phrases for the Exam for Laceration

We are going to wash (cleanse) the wound.	Vamos a lavarle (limpiarle) la herida. **Bah**-mos ah lah-**bahr**-leh (leem-pee-**ahr**-leh) lah eh-**ree**-dah.
We need to get some X rays.	Necesitamos sacarle unos rayos X. Neh-seh-see-**tah**-mos sah-**kahr**-leh **oo**-nohs **rah**-yohs **eh**-kees.

You need sutures / stitches.	Usted necesita suturas / puntadas. Oos-**tehd** neh-seh-**see**-tah soo-**too**-rahs / poon-**tah**-dahs.
I am going to give you anesthesia.	Voy a darle anestesia. **Boh**-ee ah **dahr**-leh ah-nehs-**teh**-see-ah.

Discharge Instructions for Laceration

Keep the wound clean and dry.	Mantenga limpia y seca la herida. Mahn-**tehn**-gah **leem**-pee-ah ee **seh**-kah lah eh-**ree**-dah.
Don't get the wound dirty.	No ensucie la herida. Noh ehn-**soo**-see-eh lah eh-**ree**-dah.
See your doctor in two days for a wound check.	Consulte con su médico en dos días para revisarle la herida. Kohn-**sool**-teh kohn soo **meh**-dee-koh ehn dohs **dee**-ahs **pah**-rah reh-bee-**sahr**-leh lah eh-**ree**-dah.
Your stitches should be removed in (X) days.	Hay que sacarle las puntadas en (X) días. **Ah**-ee keh sah-**kahr**-leh lahs poon-**tah**-dahs ehn (X) **dee**-ahs.
Return to the hospital (clinic) if . . .	Regrese al hospital (a la clínica) si... Reh-**greh**-seh ahl ohs-pee-**tahl** (ah lah **klee**-nee-kah) see...
you have a fever,	tiene fiebre, tee-**eh**-neh fee-**eh**-breh,

the wound becomes red,	la herida se pone roja, lah eh-**ree**-dah seh **poh**-neh **roh**-hah,
you have pus (discharge) from the wound,	tiene pus (deshecho) de la herida, tee-**eh**-neh poos (dehs-**eh**-choh) deh lah eh-**ree**-dah,
the wound swells.	se le hincha la herida. seh leh **een**-chah lah eh-**ree**-dah.

Pediatric Chief Complaints

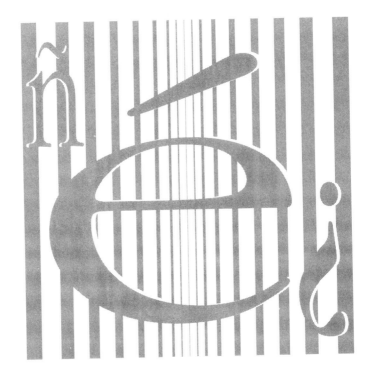

Fever

Fiebre

Fee-**eh**-breh

For how many hours or days has he / she had fever?	¿Por cuántas horas o días ha tenido fiebre? Pohr **kwahn**-tahs **oh**-rahs oh **dee**-ahs ah teh-**nee**-doh fee-**eh**-breh?
Does he / she have an earache?	¿Tiene dolor de oído? Tee-**eh**-neh doh-**lohr** deh oh-**ee**-doh?
Is he / she pulling at one or both ears?	¿Está jalándose / tirándose de una o ambas orejas? Ehs-**tah** hah-**lahn**-doh-seh / tee-**rahn**-doh-seh deh **oo**-nah oh **ahm**-bahs oh-**reh**-has?
Is he / she drinking (eating) well?	¿Está tomando (comiendo) bien? Ehs-**tah** toh-**mahn**-doh (koh-mee-**ehn**-doh) bee-**ehn**?
Does the baby sleep more than usual?	¿El / La bebé duerme más de lo normal? Ehl / Lah beh-**beh dwehr**-meh mahs deh loh nohr-**mahl**?
Does the baby cry more than usual?	¿El / La bebé llora más de lo normal? Ehl / Lah beh-**beh yoh**-rah mahs deh loh nohr-**mahl**?
Do you have difficulty waking up the child?	¿Tiene dificultad para despertar al niño (a la niña)? Tee-**eh**-neh dee-fee-kool-**tahd pah**-rah dehs-pehr-**tahr** ahl nee-nyoh (ah lah **nee**-nyah)?

Does he / she stop crying when you pick him / her up?	¿Deja de llorar cuando lo / la levanta? **Deh**-hah deh yoh-**rahr kwahn**-doh loh / lah leh-**bahn**-tah?
Has the baby been active?	¿Ha estado activo / -a el / la bebé? Ah ehs-**tah**-doh ahk-**tee**-boh / -bah ehl / lah beh-**beh**?
Does the baby smile?	¿El / La bebé sonríe? Ehl / Lah beh-**beh** sohn-**ree**-eh?
Does the baby play?	¿El / La bebé juega? Ehl / Lah beh-**beh hweh**-gah?
Have you given him / her something for the fever, such as . . .	¿Le ha dado algo para la fiebre, como... Leh ah **dah**-doh **ahl**-goh **pah**-rah lah fee-**eh**-breh, **koh**-moh...
Tylenol?	Tylenol? **Tay**-leh-nohl?
aspirin?	aspirinas? ahs-pee-**ree**-nahs?
rubbing alcohol?	frotas de alcohol? **froh**-tahs deh ahl-**kohl**?
something else?	otra cosa? **oh**-trah **koh**-sah?
When was the last time you gave him / her medicine for the fever?	¿Cuándo fue la última vez que le dio medicina para la fiebre? **Kwahn**-doh fweh lah **ool**-tee-mah behs keh leh dee-**oh** meh-dee-**see**-nah **pah**-rah lah fee-**eh**-breh?
(X) hours (days) ago.	(X) horas (días). (X) **oh**-rahs (**dee**-ahs).

Does he / she have chronic ear infections?

¿Tiene infecciones crónicas de los oídos?
Tee-**eh**-neh een-fek-see-**ohn**-ehs **kroh**-nee-kahs deh lohs oh-**ee**-dohs?

Does he / she complain of pain when he / she urinates?

¿Se queja de dolor cuando orina?
Seh **keh**-hah deh doh-**lohr kwahn**-doh oh-**ree**-nah?

Is he / she urinating more than normal?

¿Orina más de lo normal?
Oh-**ree**-nah mahs deh loh nohr-**mahl**?

Does he / she have a sore throat?

¿Tiene dolor de garganta?
Tee-**eh**-neh doh-**lohr** deh gahr-**gahn**-tah?

Is he / she drooling more than normal?

¿Babea más de lo normal?
Bah-**beh**-ah mahs deh loh nohr-**mahl**?

Does he / she have difficulty swallowing food or saliva?

¿Tiene dolor para tragar la comida o la saliva?
Tee-**eh**-neh doh-**lohr pah**-rah trah-**gahr** lah koh-**mee**-dah oh lah sah-**lee**-bah?

Does he / she have a cough?

¿Tiene tos?
Tee-**eh**-neh tohs?

Does phlegm come out when he / she coughs?

¿Le sale flema cuando tose?
Leh **sah**-leh **fleh**-mah **kwahn**-doh **toh**-seh?

What color?

¿De qué color?
Deh keh koh-**lohr**?

Is it white?

¿Es blanca?
Ehs **blahn**-kah?

Is it yellow?

¿Es amarilla?
Ehs ah-mah-**ree**-yah?

Is it green?

¿Es verde?
Ehs **behr**-deh?

Does he / she have vomiting?

¿Tiene vómito?
Tee-**eh**-neh **boh**-mee-toh?

When was the last time he / she vomited?

¿Cuándo fue la última vez que vomitó?
Kwahn-doh fweh lah **ool**-tee-mah behs keh boh-mee-**toh**?

(X) minutes (hours, days) ago.

(X) minutos (horas, días).
(X) mee-**noo**-tohs (**oh**-rahs, **dee**-ahs).

How many times a day does he / she vomit?

¿Cuántas veces vomita al día?
Kwahn-tahs **beh**-sehs boh-**mee**-tah ahl **dee**-ah?

Does he / she have diarrhea?

¿Tiene diarrea?
Tee-**eh**-neh dee-ah-**reh**-ah?

How many times a day?

¿Cuántas veces al día?
Kwahn-tahs **beh**-sehs ahl **dee**-ah?

Have you noticed blood in the diarrhea?

¿Ha notado sangre en la diarrea?
Ah noh-**tah**-doh **sahn**-greh ehn lah dee-ah-**reh**-ah?

Does he / she have pain in his / her abdomen?

¿Tiene dolor en el abdomen?
Tee-**eh**-neh doh-**lohr** ehn ehl ab-**doh**-mehn?

For how many days has he / she had abdominal pain?

¿Por cuántos días ha tenido dolor en el abdomen?
Pohr **kwahn**-tohs **dee**-ahs ah teh-**nee**-doh doh-**lohr** ehn ehl ab-**doh**-mehn?

Show me where the pain is.

Enséñeme dónde tiene el dolor.
Ehn-**sehn**-yeh-meh **dohn**-deh tee-**eh**-neh ehl doh-**lohr**.

Common Phrases for the Exam for Fever

Your baby has an ear infection.

Su bebé tiene una infección en el oído.
Soo beh-**beh** tee-**eh**-neh **oo**-nah een-fek-see-**ohn** ehn ehl oh-**ee**-doh.

Your baby has a throat infection.

Su bebé tiene una infección en la garganta.
Soo beh-**beh** tee-**eh**-neh **oo**-nah een-fek-see-**ohn** ehn lah gahr-**gahn**-tah.

Your baby has a viral infection.

Su bebé tiene una infección viral.
Soo beh-**beh** tee-**eh**-neh **oo**-nah een-fek-see-**ohn** bee-**rahl**.

Your baby has the flu.

Su bebé tiene gripe.
Soo beh-**beh** tee-**eh**-neh **gree**-peh.

Discharge Instructions for Fever

Be sure he / she drinks plenty of fluids.

Asegure que tome muchos líquidos.
Ah-seh-**goo**-reh keh **toh**-meh **moo**-chohs **lee**-kee-dohs.

Give him / her Tylenol every four hours.	Dele Tylenol cada cuatro horas. **Deh**-leh **Tay**-leh-nohl **kah**-dah koo-**ah**-troh **oh**-rahs.
Return to the hospital (clinic) if . . .	Regrese al hospital (a la clínica) si... Reh-**greh**-seh ahl ohs-pee-**tahl** (ah lah **klee**-nee-kah) see...
the fever has not gone away in two days,	no se le quita la fiebre en dos días, noh seh leh **kee**-tah lah fee-**eh**-breh ehn dohs **dee**-ahs,
he / she does not get better,	no se mejora, noh seh meh-**hoh**-rah,
or if he / she gets worse.	o se pone peor. oh seh **poh**-neh peh-**ohr**.

Earache

Dolor de Oído

Doh-**lohr** deh oh-**ee**-doh

How many days has he / she had ear pain?	¿Por cuántos días ha tenido dolor en el oído? Pohr **kwahn**-tohs **dee**-ahs ah teh-**nee**-doh doh-**lohr** ehn ehl oh-**ee**-doh?
Which ear is he / she pulling, the right or the left?	Cuál oreja está jalando, ¿la derecha o la izquierda? Kwahl oh-**reh**-hah ehs-**tah** ha-**lahn**-doh, lah deh-**reh**-chah oh lah ees-kee-**ehr**-dah?
Does he / she have a fever?	¿Tiene fiebre? Tee-**eh**-neh fee-**eh**-breh?

How many days has he / she had a fever?	¿Por cuántos días ha tenido fiebre? Pohr **kwahn**-tohs **dee**-ahs ah teh-**nee**-doh fee-**eh**-breh?
Has he / she been vomiting?	¿Tiene vómito? Tee-**eh**-neh **boh**-mee-toh?
Does he / she have diarrhea?	¿Tiene diarrea? Tee-**eh**-neh dee-ah-**reh**-ah?
Is he / she eating or taking his formula well?	¿Come o toma su fórmula bien? **Koh**-meh oh **toh**-mah soo **fohr**-moo-lah bee-**ehn**?
Is he / she crying more than normal?	¿Llora más de lo normal? **Yoh**-rah mahs deh loh nohr-**mahl**?
Is he / she sleeping more than normal?	¿Duerme más de lo normal? **Dwehr**-meh mahs deh loh nohr-**mahl**?
Can you console your baby or does he / she cry when you try to console him / her?	¿Puede consolar a su bebé o llora cuando lo / la trata de consolar? **Pweh**-deh kohn-soh-**lahr** ah soo beh-**beh** oh **yoh**-rah **kwahn**-doh loh / lah **trah**-tah deh kohn-soh-**lahr**?
Is he / she acting normally?	¿Está actuando normalmente? Ehs-**tah** ahk-too-**ahn**-doh nohr-mahl-**mehn**-teh?
Has he / she had ear infections before?	¿Ha tenido infecciones de los oídos antes? Ah teh-**nee**-doh een-fek-see-**oh**-nehs deh lohs oh-**ee**-dohs **ahn**-tehs?

Does he / she have abdominal pain?	¿Tiene dolor abdominal? Tee-**eh**-neh doh-**lohr** ab-doh-mee-**nahl**?
Is he / she allergic to penicillin?	¿Es alérgico / -a a la penicilina? Ehs ah-**lehr**-hee-koh / -kah ah lah peh-nee-see-**lee**-nah?

Common Phrases for the Exam for Earache

I am going to examine his / her ears.	Le voy a examinar los oídos. Leh **boh**-ee ah ek-sah-mee-**nahr** lohs oh-**ee**-dohs.
We need to take a rectal temperature.	Necesitamos tomarle la temperatura por el recto. Neh-seh-see-**tah**-mohs toh-**mahr**-leh lah tehm-peh-rah-**too**-rah pohr ehl **rek**-toh.
Your child has an ear infection.	Su niño / -a tiene una infección en el oído. Soo **nee**-nyoh / -nyah tee-**eh**-neh **oo**-nah een-fek-see-**ohn** ehn ehl oh-**ee**-doh.

Discharge Instructions for Earache

Give him / her the antibiotic every (X) hours.	Dele el antibiótico cada (X) horas. **Deh**-leh ehl ahn-tee-bee-**oh**-tee-koh **kah**-dah (X) **oh**-rahs.
Give him / her Tylenol every four hours if he / she is febrile.	Dele Tylenol cada cuatro horas si tiene fiebre. **Deh**-leh **Tay**-leh-nohl **kah**-dah **kwah**-troh **oh**-rahs see tee-**eh**-neh fee-**eh**-breh.

Give him / her ibuprofen every six hours.	Dele ibuprofen cada seis horas. **Deh**-leh ee-boo-**proh**-fehn **kah**-dah **seh**-ees **oh**-rahs.
Return to the hospital (clinic) if the child has . . .	Regrese al hospital (a la clínica) si el niño (la niña) tiene... Reh-**greh**-seh ahl ohs-pee-**tahl** (ah lah **klee**-nee-kah) see ehl **nee**-nyoh (lah **nee**-nyah) tee-**eh**-neh...
persistent fever,	fiebre persistente, fee-**eh**-breh pehr-sees-**tehn**-teh,
seizures,	ataques epilépticos, ah-**tah**-kehs eh-pee-**lep**-tee-kohs,
vomiting.	vómito. **boh**-mee-toh.
See your doctor in ten days to recheck the ears; sooner if the child is not better.	Consulte con su médico en diez días para revisarle los oídos; más pronto si no está mejor el niño (la niña). Kohn-**sool**-teh kohn soo **meh**-dee-koh ehn dee-**ehs dee**-ahs **pah**-rah reh-bee-**sahr**-leh lohs oh-**ee**-dohs; mahs **prohn**-toh see noh ehs-**tah** meh-**hohr**.

Vomiting

Vómito
Boh-mee-toh

How long has he / she been vomiting?	¿Por cuánto tiempo ha tenido vómito? Pohr **kwahn**-toh tee-**ehm**-poh ah teh-**nee**-doh **boh**-mee-toh?
(X) hours (days, weeks).	Por (X) horas (días, semanas). Pohr (X) **oh**-rahs (**dee**-ahs, seh-**mah**-nahs).
What color is the emesis?	¿De qué color es el vómito? Deh keh koh-**lohr** ehs ehl **boh**-mee-toh?
Is it green?	¿Es verde? Ehs **behr**-deh?
Is it yellow?	¿Es amarillo? Ehs ah-mah-**ree**-yoh?
Is it dark brown?	¿Es color café obscuro? Ehs koh-**lohr** kah-**feh** ohbs-**koo**-roh?
Is it red?	¿Es rojo? Ehs **roh**-hoh?
When he / she vomits, does the emesis shoot out in projectile form?	Cuándo vomita, ¿sale disparado el vómito en forma proyectil? **Kwahn**-doh boh-**mee**-tah, **sah**-leh dees-pah-**rah**-doh ehl **boh**-mee-toh en **fohr**-mah proh-yek-**teel**?

Does he / she vomit great quantities?	¿Vomita una gran cantidad? **Boh-mee**-tah **oo**-nah grahn kahn-tee-**dahd**?
How many times a day does he / she vomit?	¿Cuántas veces vomita al día? **Kwahn**-tahs **beh**-sehs boh-**mee**-tah ahl **dee**-ah?
When was the last time he / she vomited?	¿Cuándo fue la última vez que vomitó? **Kwahn**-doh fweh lah **ool**-tee-mah behs keh boh-mee-**toh**?
(X) minutes (hours, days) ago.	(X) minutos (horas, días). (X) mee-**noo**-tohs (**oh**-rahs, **dee**-ahs).
Has the baby lost weight?	¿Ha perdido peso el / la bebé? Ah pehr-**dee**-doh **peh**-soh ehl / lah beh-**beh**?
How many pounds?	¿Cuántas libras? **Kwahn**-tahs **lee**-brahs?
Does he / she have diarrhea?	¿Tiene diarrea? Tee-**eh**-neh dee-ah-**reh**-ah?
How many times a day does he / she have diarrhea?	¿Cuántas veces al día tiene diarrea? **Kwahn**-tahs **beh**-sehs ahl **dee**-ah tee-**eh**-neh dee-ah-**reh**-ah?
Have you noticed blood in the diarrhea?	¿Ha notado sangre en la diarrea? Ah noh-**tah**-doh **sahn**-greh ehn lah dee-ah-**reh**-ah?
Have you recently traveled outside the country?	¿Recientemente ha viajado fuera del país? Reh-see-ehn-teh-**mehn**-teh ah bee-ah-**hah**-doh **fweh**-rah dehl pah-**ees**?

To where?

¿A dónde?
Ah **dohn**-deh?

Does he / she have a fever?

¿Tiene fiebre?
Tee-**eh**-neh fee-**eh**-breh?

Does the child vomit immediately after feeding him / her formula?

¿Vomita el niño / la niña inmediatamente después de tomar su fórmula?
Boh-**mee**-tah ehl **nee**-nyoh / lah **nee**-nyah een-meh-dee-ah-tah-**mehn**-teh dehs-**pwehs** deh toh-**mahr** soo **fohr**-moo-lah?

Does it seem like he / she is hungry?

¿Le parece que tiene hambre?
Leh pah-**reh**-seh keh tee-**eh**-neh **ahm**-breh?

Have you changed his / her formula?

¿Le ha cambiado la fórmula?
Leh ah kahm-bee-**ah**-doh lah **fohr**-moo-lah?

What brand of formula does he / she take?

¿Qué marca de fórmula toma?
Keh **mahr**-kah deh **fohr**-moo-lah **toh**-mah?

Do you give him / her cow's milk?

¿Le da leche de vaca?
Leh dah **leh**-cheh deh **bah**-kah?

Does the baby vomit only when you give him / her milk?

¿El / La bebé vomita solamente cuándo le da leche?
Ehl / Lah beh-**beh** boh-**mee**-tah soh-lah-**mehn**-teh **kwahn**-doh leh dah **leh**-cheh?

Is there another person in the house with the same symptoms?

¿Hay otra persona en casa con los mismos síntomas?
Ah-ee **oh**-trah pehr-**soh**-nah ehn **kah**-sah kohn lohs **mees**-mohs **seen**-toh-mahs?

Does the baby make tears when he / she cries?	Cuándo el / la bebé llora, ¿le salen lágrimas? **Kwahn**-doh ehl / lah beh-**beh yoh**-rah, leh **sah**-lehn **lah**-gree-mahs?
When was the last time he / she urinated?	¿Cuándo fue la última vez que orinó? **Kwahn**-doh fweh lah **ool**-tee-mah behs keh oh-**ree**-noh?

Common Phrases for the Exam for Vomiting

We need to do blood and urine tests.	Necesitamos hacerle análisis de sangre y orina. Neh-seh-see-**tah**-mos ah-**sehr**-leh ah-**nah**-lee-sees deh **sahn**-greh ee oh-**ree**-nah.
Your baby is dehydrated.	Su bebé está deshidratado / -a. Soo beh-**beh** ehs-**tah** dehs-ee-drah-**tah**-doh / -dah.
Your baby needs an IV.	Su bebé necesita suero intravenoso. Soo beh-**beh** neh-seh-**see**-tah soo-**eh**-roh een-trah-beh-**noh**-soh.
We are going to admit the baby.	Vamos a internar al bebé. **Bah**-mohs ah een-tehr-**nahr** ahl beh-**beh**.

Discharge Instructions for Vomiting

Don't give the baby cow's milk for a day.	No le de leche de vaca al bebé por un día. Noh leh deh **leh**-cheh deh **bah**-kah ahl beh-**beh** pohr oon **dee**-ah.

Give him / her Pedialyte for a day.	Dele Pedialyte por un día. **Deh**-leh Pee-dee-ah-**lah**-eet pohr oon **dee**-ah.
Return to the hospital (clinic) if your baby . . .	Regrese al hospital (a la clínica) si su bebé... Reh-**greh**-seh ahl ohs-pee-**tahl** (ah lah **klee**-nee-kah) see soo beh-**beh**...
continues vomiting,	sigue vomitando, **see**-geh boh-mee-**tahn**-doh,
has a fever,	tiene fiebre, tee-**eh**-neh fee-**eh**-breh,
stops making tears or urine.	deja de hacer lágrimas u orina. **deh**-hah deh ah-**sehr lah**-gree-mahs oo oh-**ree**-nah.

Shortness of Breath or Asthma

Falta de Aire o Asma

Fahl-tah deh **ah**-ee-reh oh **ahs**-mah

How many days (weeks) has he / she had trouble breathing?	¿Por cuántos días (Por cuántas semanas) ha tenido dificultad para respirar? Pohr **kwahn**-tohs **dee**-ahs (Pohr **kwahn**-tahs seh-**mah**-nahs) ah teh-**nee**-doh dee-fee-kool-**tahd pah**-rah rehs-pee-**rahr**?
Does he / she have a cough?	¿Tiene tos? Tee-**eh**-neh tohs?

When did the cough start?	¿Cuándo empezó la tos? **Kwahn**-doh ehm-peh-**soh** lah tohs?
(X) hours (days, weeks) ago.	(X) horas (días, semanas). (X) **oh**-rahs (**dee**-ahs, seh-**mah**-nahs).
Does he / she have phlegm when he / she coughs?	¿Le sale flema cuando tose? Leh **sah**-leh **fleh**-mah **kwahn**-doh **toh**-seh?
What color is the phlegm?	¿De qué color es la flema? Deh keh koh-**lohr** ehs lah **fleh**-mah?
Is it white?	¿Es blanca? Ehs **blahn**-kah?
Is it yellow?	¿Es amarilla? Ehs ah-mah-**ree**-yah?
Is it green?	¿Es verde? Ehs **behr**-deh?
Do you believe the baby inhaled something (such as a toy or a peanut)?	¿Usted cree que el / la bebé aspiró algo (como un juguete o un cacahuate)? Oos-**tehd kreh**-eh keh ehl / lah beh-**beh** ahs-pee-**roh ahl**-goh (**koh**-moh oon hoo-**geh**-teh oh oon kah-kah-**hwah**-teh)?
Does he / she have a fever?	¿Tiene fiebre? Tee-**eh**-neh fee-**eh**-breh?
How long has he / she had a fever?	¿Por cuánto tiempo ha tenido fiebre? Pohr **kwahn**-toh tee-**ehm**-poh ah teh-**nee**-doh fee-**eh**-breh?

(X) hours (days, weeks).	Por (X) horas (días, semanas). Pohr (X) **oh**-rahs (**dee**-ahs, seh-**mah**-nahs).
Does he / she have a history of asthma?	¿Tiene una historia de asma? Tee-**eh**-neh **oo**-nah ees-**toh**-ree-ah deh **ahs**-mah?
What medicine does he / she take?	Qué medicina toma? Keh meh-dee-**see**-nah **toh**-mah?
Ventolin?	¿Ventolina? Behn-toh-**lee**-nah?
Theodur?	¿Theodur? Teh-oh-**duhr**?
Prednisone?	¿Prednisona? Prehd-nee-**soh**-nah?
Azmacort?	¿Azmacort? Ahs-mah-**kohrt**?
How many times a day does he / she take the medicine?	¿Cuántas veces al día toma la medicina? Kwahn-tahs **beh**-sehs ahl **dee**-ah **toh**-mah lah meh-dee-**see**-nah?
When was the last time he / she took the medicine?	¿Cuándo fue la última vez que tomó la medicina? **Kwahn**-doh fweh lah **ool**-tee-mah behs keh toh-**moh** lah meh-dee-**see**-nah?
(X) hours (days, weeks) ago.	(X) horas (días, semanas). (X) **oh**-rahs (**dee**-ahs, seh-**mah**-nahs).

Do you think that his /
her condition worsened
because of . . .

¿Piensa usted que su
condición empeoró por...
Pee-**ehn**-sah oos-**tehd** keh
soo kohn-dee-see-**ohn**
ehm-peh-oh-**roh** pohr...

a change in the
environment or
weather?

un cambio del
ambiente o clima?
oon **kahm**-bee-oh
dehl ahm-bee-**ehn**-teh
oh **klee**-mah?

dust?

polvo?
pohl-boh?

cigarette smoke?

humo de cigarillo?
oo-moh deh see-gah-
ree-yoh?

running (exercise)?

correr (hacer
ejercicio)?
koh-**rehr** (ah-**sehr** eh-
her-**see**-see-oh)?

How many times has
he / she been hospitalized
for asthma attacks?

¿Cuántas veces ha sido
hospitalizado / -a por
ataques de asma?
Kwahn-tahs **beh**-sehs ah
see-doh ohs-pee-tah-lee-
sah-doh / -dah pohr ah-
tah-kehs deh **ahs**-mah?

Does he / she make noise
when he / she breathes?

¿Hace ruido cuándo respira?
Ah-seh roo-**ee**-doh **kwahn**-doh
rehs-**pee**-rah?

Does his / her chest wheeze
or have a whistling sound?

¿Le chifla o tiene silbido el
pecho?
Leh **chee**-flah oh tee-**eh**-neh
seel-**bee**-doh ehl **peh**-choh?

Does he / she have a hoarse sound in his / her chest?	¿Tiene un sonido ronco en el pecho? Tee-**eh**-neh oon soh-**nee**-doh **ron**-koh ehn ehl **peh**-choh?

Common Phrases for the Exam for Shortness of Breath or Asthma

We need to do an X ray of his / her chest.	Necesitamos hacerle una radiografía del pecho. Neh-seh-see-**tah**-mohs ah-**sehr**-leh **oo**-nah rah-dee-oh-grah-**fee**-ah dehl **peh**-choh.
Your child needs treatment.	Su niño / -a necesita tratamiento. Soo **nee**-nyoh / -nyah neh-seh-**see**-tah trah-tah-mee-**ehn**-toh.
Your child needs an IV.	Su niño / -a necesita suero intravenoso. Soo **nee**-nyoh / -nyah neh-seh-**see**-tah soo-**eh**-roh een-trah-beh-**noh**-soh.
Your child has pneumonia.	Su niño / -a tiene pulmonía. Soo **nee**-nyoh / -nyah tee-**eh**-neh pool-moh-**nee**-ah.
Your child has asthma.	Su niño / -a tiene asma. Soo **nee**-nyoh / -nyah tee-**eh**-neh **ahs**-mah.
Your child has the flu.	Su niño / -a tiene gripe. Soo **nee**-nyoh / -nyah tee-**eh**-neh **gree**-peh.

Discharge Instructions for Shortness of Breath or Asthma

Take the medications as indicated.

Tome las medicinas como le indicaron.
Toh-meh lahs meh-dee-**see**-nahs **koh**-moh leh een-dee-**kah**-rohn.

Return to the hospital (clinic) if your baby . . .

Regrese al hospital (a la clínica) si su bebé...
Reh-**greh**-seh ahl ohs-pee-**tahl** (ah lah **klee**-nee-kah) see soo beh-**beh**...

is still short of breath,

sigue con falta de aire,
see-geh kohn **fahl**-tah deh **ah**-ee-reh,

has a fever,

tiene fiebre,
tee-**eh**-neh fee-**eh**-breh,

has vomiting,

tiene vómito,
tee-**eh**-neh **boh**-mee-toh,

is not getting better.

no mejora.
noh meh-**hoh**-rah.

Abdominal Pain

Dolor Abdominal

Doh-**lohr** ab-**doh**-mee-nahl

Show me where the pain started.

Enséñeme dónde empezó el dolor.
Ehn-**seh**-nyeh-meh **dohn**-deh ehm-peh-**soh** ehl doh-**lohr**.

Show me with one finger where he / she has the pain.	Enséñeme con un solo dedo dónde tiene el dolor. Ehn-**seh**-nyeh-meh kohn oon **soh**-loh **deh**-doh **dohn**-deh tee-**eh**-neh ehl doh-**lohr**.
How long has he / she had pain?	¿Por cuánto tiempo ha tenido dolor? Pohr **kwahn**-toh tee-**ehm**-poh ah teh-**nee**-doh ehl doh-**lohr**?
For (X) hours (days, weeks).	Por (X) horas (días, semanas). Pohr (X) **oh**-rahs (**dee**-ahs, seh-**mah**-nahs).
Is the pain constant?	¿Es el dolor constante? Ehs ehl doh-**lohr** kohns-**tahn**-teh?
Does the pain come and go?	¿Le va y viene el dolor? Leh bah ee bee-**eh**-neh ehl doh-**lohr**?
Does the pain go to his / her back?	¿Le viaja el dolor a la espalda? Leh bee-**ah**-hah ehl doh-**lohr** ah lah ehs-**pahl**-dah?
Does the pain go to his testicles?	¿Le viaja el dolor a los testículos? Leh bee-**ah**-hah ehl doh-**lohr** ah lohs tehs-**tee**-koo-lohs?
Does the pain go to the groin?	¿Le viaja el dolor a la ingle? Leh bee-**ah**-hah ehl doh-**lohr** ah lah **een**-gleh?
Does the pain go to his / her bladder?	¿Le viaja el dolor a la vejiga? Leh bee-**ah**-hah ehl doh-**lohr** ah lah beh-**hee**-gah?
Does he / she have vomiting?	¿Tiene vómito? Tee-**eh**-neh **boh**-mee-toh?

Did the vomiting or the pain start first?	¿Empezó primero el vómito o el dolor? Ehm-peh-**soh** pree-**meh**-roh ehl **boh**-mee-toh oh ehl doh-**lohr**?
How many times has he / she vomited today?	¿Cuántas veces ha vomitado hoy? **Kwahn**-tahs **beh**-sehs ah boh-mee-**tah**-doh **oh**-ee?
Does he / she have diarrhea?	¿Tiene diarrea? Tee-**eh**-neh dee-ah-**reh**-ah?
How many times today?	¿Cuántas veces hoy? **Kwahn**-tahs **beh**-sehs oh-ee?
When was the last time he / she urinated (had a bowel movement)?	¿Cuándo fue la última vez que orinó (obró / defecó)? **Kwahn**-doh fweh lah **ool**-tee-mah behs keh oh-ree-**noh** (oh-**broh** / deh-feh-**koh**)?
Does he / she have a fever?	¿Tiene fiebre? Tee-**eh**-neh fee-**eh**-breh?
How long has he / she had a fever?	¿Por cuánto tiempo ha tenido fiebre? Pohr **kwahn**-toh tee-**ehm**-poh ah teh-**nee**-doh fee-**eh**-breh?
(X) hours (days, weeks).	Por (X) horas (días, semanas). Pohr (X) **oh**-rahs (**dee**-ahs, seh-**mah**-nahs).
Does he / she complain of pain upon urinating?	¿Se queja de dolor cuando orina? Seh **keh**-hah deh doh-**lohr** **kwahn**-doh oh-**ree**-nah?

When was the last time he / she ate?	¿Cuándo fue la última vez que comió? **Kwahn**-doh fweh lah **ool**-tee-mah behs keh koh-mee-**oh**?
Is your child hungry?	¿Tiene hambre su hijo / -a? Tee-**eh**-neh **ahm**-breh soo **ee**-hoh / -hah?
Does he / she have a cough?	¿Tiene tos? Tee-**eh**-neh tohs?
Does he / she have a sore throat?	¿Tiene dolor de garganta? Tee-**eh**-neh doh-**lohr** deh gahr-**gahn**-tah?

Common Phrases for the Exam for Abdominal Pain

I need to examine his / her abdomen.	Necesito examinarle el abdomen. Neh-seh-**see**-toh ek-sah-mee-**nahr**-leh ehl ab-**doh**-mehn.
Your child has appendicitis.	Su hijo / -a tiene apendicitis. Soo **ee**-hoh / -hah tee-**eh**-neh ah-pehn-dee-see-tees.
Your child needs an operation.	Su hijo / -a necesita una operacion. Soo **ee**-hoh / -hah neh-seh-**see**-tah **oo**-nah oh-peh-rah-see-**ohn**.
Your child has a viral infection.	Su hijo / -a tiene infeccion viral. Soo **ee**-hoh / -hah tee-**eh**-neh een-fek-see-**ohn** bee-**rahl**.

Your child needs intravenous fluids.

Su hijo / -a necesita liquidos intravenosos (suero).
Soo **ee**-hoh / -hah neh-seh-**see**-tah **lee**-kee-dohs een-trah-beh-**noh**-sohs (**sweh**-roh).

We need to do blood and urine tests.

Necesitamos hacerle pruebas de sangre y orina.
Neh-seh-see-**tah**-mohs ah-**sehr**-leh prweh-bahs deh **sahn**-greh ee oh-**ree**-nah.

Discharge Instructions for Abdominal Pain

Return to the hospital (clinic) if . . .

Regrese al hospital (a la clínica) si...
Reh-**greh**-seh ahl ohs-pee-**tahl** (ah lah **klee**-nee-kah) see...

your child has a fever,

su hijo / -a tiene fiebre,
soo **ee**-hoh / -hah tee-**eh**-neh fee-**eh**-breh,

your child is vomiting,

su hijo / -a tiene vómito,
soo **ee**-hoh / -hah tee-**eh**-neh **boh**-mee-toh,

the pain is worse (increases).

el dolor se pone peor (aumenta).
ehl doh-**lohr** seh **poh**-neh peh-**ohr** (ah-oo-**mehn**-tah).

Seizures

Convulsiones o Ataques Epilepticos

Kohn-bool-see-**ohn**-ehs oh ah-**tah**-kehs eh-**pee**-lep-tee-kos

When did the convulsion occur?

¿Cuándo le ocurrió la convulsión?
Kwahn-doh leh oh-koo-ree-**oh** lah kohn-bool-see-**ohn**?

(X) hours (days) ago.

(X) horas (días).
(X) **oh**-rahs (**dee**-ahs).

What was the attack like?

¿Cómo fue el ataque?
Koh-moh fweh ehl ah-**tah**-keh?

Was it a general seizure?

¿Fue una convulsión general?
Fweh **oo**-nah kohn-bool-see-**ohn** heh-neh-**rahl**?

Was it a seizure of one part of the body?

¿Fue una convulsión en una sola parte del cuerpo?
Fweh **oo**-nah kohn-bool-see-**ohn** ehn **oo**-nah **soh**-lah **pahr**-teh dehl **kwehr**-poh?

Was it the right (left) arm?

¿Fue en el brazo derecho (izquierdo)?
Fweh ehn ehl **brah**-soh deh-**reh**-choh (ees-kee-**ehr**-doh)?

Was it the right (left) leg?

¿Fue en la pierna derecha (izquierda)?
Fweh ehn lah pee-**ehr**-nah deh-**reh**-chah (ees-kee-**ehr**-dah)?

Was it the face?	¿Fue en la cara? Fweh ehn lah **kah**-rah?
Did the child stop breathing and turn pale and limp?	¿Dejó de respirar el niño / la niña y se puso pálido y sin fuerza? Deh-**hoh** deh rehs-pee-**rahr** ehl **nee**-nyoh / lah **nee**-nyah, ee seh **poo**-soh **pah**-lee-doh ee seen **fwehr**-sah?
Did the child stop breathing and turn blue and stiff?	¿Dejó de respirar el niño / la niña y se puso morado / -a y tieso / -a? Deh-**hoh** deh rehs-pee-**rahr** ehl **nee**-nyoh / lah **nee**-nyah ee seh **poo**-soh moh-**rah**-doh / -dah ee tee-**eh**-soh / -sah?
Did he / she turn stiff (rigid) with the attack?	¿Se puso tieso (rígido) con el ataque? Seh **poo**-soh tee-**eh**-soh (**ree**-hee-doh) kohn ehl ah-**tah**-keh?
Did he / she turn limp (flaccid) and weak with the attack?	¿Se puso flojo (fláccido) y débil con el ataque? Seh **poo**-soh **floh**-hoh (**flah**-see-doh) ee **deh**-beel kohn ehl ah-**tah**-keh?
Was the seizure provoked by a scolding, anger, or an upset?	¿El ataque fue provocado por un regaño, enojo, o disgusto? Ehl ah-**tah**-keh fweh proh-boh-**kah**-doh pohr oon reh-**gah**-nyoh, eh-**noh**-hoh, oh dees-**goos**-toh?
Did the child lose consciousness?	¿Perdió el niño / la niña el conocimiento? Pehr-dee-**oh** ehl **nee**-nyoh / lah **nee**-nyah ehl koh-noh-see-mee-**ehn**-toh?

After the convulsion, did he / she remain asleep or unconscious?	Después de la convulsión, ¿permaneció dormido / -a o inconsciente? Dehs-**pwehs** deh lah kohn-bool-see-**ohn,** pehr-mah-neh-see-**oh** dohr-**mee**-doh / -dah oh een-kohn-see-**ehn**-teh?
Did he / she regain consciousness rapidly or slowly?	¿Recobró el conocimiento rápidamente o lentamente? Reh-koh-**broh** ehl koh-noh-see-mee-**ehn**-toh rah-pee-dah-**mehn**-teh oh lehn-tah-**mehn**-teh?
How long did the convulsion last?	¿Cuánto tiempo duró la convulsión? **Kwahn**-toh tee-**ehm**-poh doo-**roh** lah kohn-bool-see-**ohn?**
More than 15 minutes?	¿Más de 15 minutos? Mahs deh **keen**-seh mee-**noo**-tohs?
Less than 15 minutes?	¿Menos de 15 minutos? **Meh**-nohs deh **keen**-seh mee-**noo**-tohs?
Did he / she have a fever before the attack?	¿Tenía fiebre antes de darle el ataque? Teh-**nee**-ah fee-**eh**-breh **ahn**-tehs deh **dahr**-leh ehl ah-**tah**-keh?
Has he / she had more than one attack in 24 hours?	¿Ha tenido más de un ataque en 24 horas? Ah teh-**nee**-doh mahs deh oon ah-**tah**-keh ehn **beh**-een-tee-**kwah**-troh **oh**-rahs?

Has he / she ever had attacks like this?	¿Alguna vez ha tenido ataques como éste? Ahl-**goo**-nah behs ah teh-**nee**-doh ah-**tah**-kehs **koh**-moh **ehs**-teh?
Have they ever told you that the child has epilepsy?	¿Alguna vez le han dicho que el niño / la niña tiene epilepsia? Ahl-**goo**-nah behs leh ahn **dee**-choh keh ehl **nee**-nyoh / lah **nee**-nyah tee-**eh**-neh eh-pee-**lep**-see-ah?
Has he / she hit his / her head recently?	¿Se ha golpeado la cabeza recientemente? Seh ah gohl-peh-**ah**-doh lah kah-**beh**-sah reh-see-ehn-teh-**mehn**-teh?
Was your child born premature?	¿Nació su hijo / -a prematuro / -a? Nah-see-**oh** soo **ee**-hoh / -hah preh-mah-**too**-roh / -rah?
At how many weeks or months was he / she born?	¿A cuántas semanas o meses nació? Ah **kwahn**-tahs seh-**mah**-nahs oh **meh**-sehs nah-see-**oh**?
Does he / she have a problem with his / her brain?	¿Tiene algún problema con el cerebro? Tee-**eh**-neh ahl-**goon** proh-**bleh**-mah kohn ehl seh-**reh**-broh?
Is he / she mentally retarded?	¿Tiene retraso mental? Tee-**eh**-neh reh-**trah**-soh mehn-**tahl**?

Does he / she have a family member with epilepsy?	¿Tiene algún familiar con epilepsia? Tee-**eh**-neh ahl-**goon** fah-mee-lee-**ahr** kohn eh-pee-**lep**-see-ah?
The child's mother (father)?	¿El padre (la madre) del niño (de la niña)? Ehl **pah**-dreh (lah **mah**-dreh) dehl **nee**-nyoh (deh lah **nee**-nyah)?
A sibling?	¿Algún hermano del niño (de la niña)? Ahl-**goon** ehr-**mah**-noh dehl **nee**-nyoh (deh lah **nee**-nyah)?
Someone else?	¿Otra persona? **Oh**-trah pehr-**soh**-nah?
Does he / she have a family member that has seizures when febrile?	¿Tiene algún familiar a quien le den ataques cuándo tiene fiebre? Tee-**eh**-neh ahl-**goon** fah-mee-lee-**ahr** ah kee-**ehn** leh dehn ah-**tah**-kehs **kwahn**-doh tee-**eh**-neh fee-**eh**-breh?
The child's mother (father)?	¿El padre (la madre) del niño (de la niña)? Ehl **pah**-dreh (lah **mah**-dreh) dehl **nee**-nyoh (deh lah **nee**-nyah)?
A sibling?	¿Algún hermano del niño (de la niña)? Ahl-**goon** ehr-**mah**-noh dehl **nee**-nyoh (deh lah **nee**-nyah)?
Someone else?	¿Otra persona? **Oh**-trah pehr-**soh**-nah?

Is the child taking medication?	¿Toma medicina el niño / la niña? **Toh**-mah meh-dee-**see**-nah ehl **nee**-nyoh / lah **nee**-nyah?
Did you notice if he / she took pills of yours or some relative?	¿No se ha dado cuenta si tomó algunas pastillas de usted o de algún familiar? Noh seh ah **dah**-doh **kwehn**-tah see toh-**moh** ahl-**goo**-nahs pahs-**tee**-yahs deh oos-**tehd** oh deh ahl-**goon** fah-mee-lee-**ahr**?
Does he / she have a fever?	¿Tiene fiebre? Tee-**eh**-neh fee-**eh**-breh?
Does he / she have the flu or a cold?	¿Tiene gripe o catarro? Tee-**eh**-neh **gree**-peh oh kah-**tah**-roh?
Has he / she been vomiting?	¿Tiene vómito? Tee-**eh**-neh **boh**-mee-toh?
Does he / she have diarrhea?	¿Tiene diarrea? Tee-**eh**-neh dee-ah-**reh**-ah?
Have you given him / her aspirin or Tylenol?	¿Le ha dado aspirinas o Tylenol? Le ah **dah**-doh ahs-pee-**ree**-nahs oh **Tay**-leh-nohl?
How many drops (teaspoons, tablets)?	¿Cuántas gotas (cucharitas, pastillas)? **Kwahn**-tahs **goh**-tahs (koo-cha-**ree**-tahs, pahs-**tee**-yahs)?
Every how many hours?	¿Cada cuántas horas? **Kah**-dah **kwahn**-tahs **oh**-rahs?

Have you rubbed your child with alcohol?	¿Ha frotado a su hijo / -a con alcohol? Ah froh-**tah**-doh ah soo **ee**-hoh / -hah kohn ahl-**kohl**?
Has he / she been eating well?	¿Ha estado comiendo bien? Ah ehs-**tah**-doh koh-mee-**ehn**-doh bee-**ehn**?
Has anybody else in the family been sick?	¿Alguien más en la familia ha estado enfermo? **Ahl**-gee-ehn mahs ehn lah fah-**mee**-lee-ah ah ehs-**tah**-doh ehn-**fehr**-moh?
Was he / she acting normal before the seizure?	¿Estaba actuando normal antes del ataque? Ehs-**tah**-bah ahk-too-**ahn**-doh nohr-**mahl ahn**-tehs dehl ah-**tah**-keh?
Was he / she sleeping more than usual before the seizure?	¿Dormía más de lo usual antes del ataque? Dohr-**mee**-ah mahs deh loh oo-soo-**ahl ahn**-tehs dehl ah-**tah**-keh?
Was he / she more fussy than usual before the seizure?	¿Estaba más molesto / -a de lo usual antes del ataque? Ehs-**tah**-bah mahs moh-**lehs**-toh / -tah deh loh oo-soo-**ahl ahn**-tehs dehl ah-**tah**-keh?
Did you have problems consoling him / her today?	¿Tuvo problemas al consolarlo / la hoy? **Too**-boh proh-**bleh**-mahs ahl kohn-soh-**lahr**-loh / -lah **oh**-ee?

Common Phrases for the Exam for Seizures

Your child needs a CT scan of the brain.

Su hijo / a necesita un CT (una tomografía) del cerebro.
Soo **ee**-hoh / -hah neh-seh-**see**-tah oon seh-teh (**oo**-nah toh-moh-grah-**fee**-ah) dehl seh-**reh**-broh.

I need to do a lumbar puncture.

Necesito hacerle una punción lumbar.
Neh-seh-**see**-toh ah-**sehr**-leh **oo**-nah poon-see-**ohn** loom-**bahr.**

I am going to put a needle in his / her back to draw some fluid that surrounds the brain.

Voy a ponerle una aguja en la espalda para sacarle líquido que rodea al cerebro.
Boh-ee ah poh-**neh**-leh **oo**-nah ah-**goo**-hah ehn lah **ehs**-pahl-dah **pah**-rah sah-**kahr**-leh lee-**kee**-doh **keh** roh-**deh**-ah ahl seh-**reh**-broh.

Your child has a brain infection (meningitis).

Su hijo / -a tiene una infección en el cerebro (meningitis).
Soo **ee**-hoh / -hah tee-**eh**-neh **oo**-nah een-fek-see-**ohn** ehn ehl seh-**reh**-broh (meh-neen-**hee**-tees).

Your child had the seizure because of the fever.

Su hijo / -a tuvo el ataque por la fiebre.
Soo **ee**-hoh / -hah **too**-boh ehl ah-**tah**-keh pohr lah fee-**yeh**-breh.

We need to admit him / her.

Necesitamos internarlo / la.
Neh-seh-see-**tah**-mohs een-ter-**nahr**-loh / -lah.

Discharge Instructions for Seizures

Return to the hospital (clinic) if your child . . .	Regrese al hospital (a la clínica) si su hijo / -a... Reh-**greh**-seh ahl ohs-pee-**tahl** (ah lah **klee**-nee-kah) see soo **ee**-hoh / -hah...
continues to have seizures,	continúa teniendo ataques epilépticos, kohn-tee-**noo**-ah teh-nee-**ehn**-doh ah-**tah**-kehs eh-pee-**lep**-tee-kohs,
has trouble walking or talking,	tiene problemas al caminar o hablar, tee-**eh**-neh proh-**bleh**-mahs ahl kah-mee-**nahr** oh ah-**blahr**,
doesn't have any more seizure medication.	no tiene más medicina para los ataques epilépticos. noh tee-**eh**-neh mahs meh-dee-**see**-nah **pah**-rah lohs ah-**tah**-kehs eh-pee-**lep**-tee-kohs.

Rash

Erupción

Eh-roop-see-**ohn**

When did the rash appear?	¿Cuándo empezó la erupción? **Kwahn**-doh ehm-peh-**soh** lah eh-roop-see-**ohn**?
(When did the hives [spots] appear?)	(¿Cuándo empezaron las ronchas [manchas]?) (**Kwahn**-doh ehm-peh-**sah**-rohn lahs **rohn**-chahs [**mahn**-chahs]?)

(X) hours (days, weeks) ago.	(X) horas (días, semanas). (X) **oh**-rahs (**dee**-ahs, seh-**mah**-nahs).
Has the baby had something like this before?	¿Ha tenido algo así antes el / la bebé? Ah teh-**nee**-doh **ahl**-goh ah-**see ahn**-tehs ehl / lah beh-**beh**?
Where did the rash begin?	¿Dónde empezó la erupción? **Dohn**-deh ehm-peh-**soh** lah eh-roop-see-**ohn**?
(Where did the hives [spots] begin?)	(¿Dónde empezaron las ronchas [manchas]?) (**Dohn**-deh ehm-peh-**sah**-rohn lahs **rohn**-chahs [**mahn**-chahs]?)
On his / her face?	¿En la cara? Ehn lah **kah**-rah?
On his / her chest?	¿En el pecho? Ehn ehl **peh**-choh?
On his / her legs?	¿En las piernas? Ehn lahs pee-**ehr**-nahs?
On his / her arms?	¿En los brazos? Ehn lohs **brah**-sohs?
Does he / she have a fever?	¿Tiene fiebre? Tee-**eh**-neh fee-**eh**-breh?
Does the baby have itching?	¿Tiene comezón el / la bebé? Tee-**eh**-neh koh-meh-**sohn** ehl / lah beh-**beh**?
Is the baby's voice hoarse?	¿Tiene la voz ronca el / la bebé? Tee-**eh**-neh lah bohs **rohn**-kah ehl / lah beh-**beh**?

Does he / she have trouble breathing?	¿Tiene problemas al respirar? Tee-**eh**-neh proh-**bleh**-mahs ahl rehs-pee-**rahr**?
Is there wheezing in his / her chest?	¿Le chifla el pecho? Leh **chee**-flah ehl **peh**-choh?
Is he / she taking any medication?	¿Está tomando alguna medicina? Ehs-**tah** toh-**mahn**-doh ahl-**goo**-nah meh-dee-**see**-nah?
Antibiotics?	¿Antibióticos? Ahn-tee-bee-**oh**-tee-kohs?
Something else?	¿Otra medicina? **Oh**-trah meh-dee-**see**-nah?
Do you have a new dog or cat at home?	¿Tienen un nuevo perro o gato en casa? Tee-**eh**-nehn oon **nweh**-boh **peh**-roh oh **gah**-toh ehn **kah**-sah?
Have you used a new soap, shampoo, detergent, or lotion?	¿Ha usado un nuevo jabón, champú, detergente, o loción? Ah oo-**sah**-doh oon **nweh**-boh hah-**bohn**, chahm-**poo**, deh-tehr-**hehn**-teh, oh loh-see-**ohn**?
Did you give him / her a new food?	¿Le dio alguna comida nueva? Leh dee-**oh** ahl-**goo**-nah koh-**mee**-dah **nweh**-bah?
Have you changed his / her formula?	¿Le ha cambiado la formula? Leh ah kahm-bee-**ah**-doh lah **fohr**-moo-lah?
Did you give the child Benadryl?	¿Le dio Benadryl al niño (a la niña)? Leh dee-**oh** Beh-nah-**dreel** ahl **nee**-nyoh (ah lah **nee**-nyah)?

Are your child's shots up to date?	¿Está al corriente con sus vacunas su hijo / -a? Ehs-**tah** ahl koh-ree-**ehn**-teh kohn soos bah-**koo**-nahs soo **ee**-hoh / -hah?
Does the baby have allergies?	¿Tiene alergias el / la bebé? Tee-**eh**-neh ah-**lehr**-hee-ahs ehl / lah beh-**beh**?

Common Phrases for the Exam for Rash

Your baby has an allergic reaction.	Su bebé tiene una reacción alérgica. Soo beh-**beh** tee-**eh**-neh **oo**-nah reh-ahk-see-**ohn** ah-**lehr**-hee-kah.
Your baby has a viral infection.	Su bebé tiene una infección viral. Soo beh-**beh** tee-**eh**-neh **oo**-nah een-fek-see-**ohn** bee-**rahl**.
Your baby has chicken pox.	Su bebé tiene varicela (viruelas locas). Soo beh-**beh** tee-**eh**-neh bah-ree-**seh**-lah (bee-roo-**eh**-lahs loh-kahs).
Your baby has the measles.	Su bebé tiene sarampión. Soo beh-**beh** tee-**eh**-neh sah-rahm-pee-**ohn**.

Discharge Instructions for Rash

Stop using the new soap (shampoo, cream, detergent).	Deje de usar el nuevo jabón (champú, crema, detergente). **Deh**-heh deh oo-**sahr** ehl **nweh**-boh hah-**bohn** (chahm-**poo**, **kreh**-mah, deh-tehr-**hehn**-teh).

(*if allergic to an antibiotic*) Stop using the antibiotic.	Deje de usar el antibiótico. **Deh**-heh deh oo-**sahr** ehl ahn-tee-bee-**oh**-tee-koh.
Give your child Benadryl every six hours.	Dele Benadryl a su niño / -a cada seis horas. **Deh**-leh Beh-nah-**dreel** ah soo **nee**-nyoh / -nyah **kah**-dah **seh**-ees **oh**-rahs.
Return to the hospital (clinic) if . . .	Regrese al hospital (a la clínica) si... Reh-**greh**-seh ahl ohs-pee-**tahl** (ah lah **klee**-nee-kah) see...
the child is short of breath,	el niño (la niña) tiene falta de aire, ehl **nee**-nyoh (lah **nee**-nyah) tee-**eh**-neh **fahl**-tah deh **ah**-ee-reh,
there is wheezing in his / her chest,	le chifla el pecho, leh **chee**-flah ehl **peh**-choh,
his / her body swells up,	se le hincha el cuerpo, seh leh **een**-chah ehl **kwehr**-poh,
or the rash worsens.	o la erupción está peor. oh lah eh-roop-see-**ohn** ehs-**tah** peh-**ohr**.

Crying or Colic

Llorando o Cólico

Yoh-rahn-doh oh **koh**-lee-koh

When did the baby start crying?	¿Cuándo empezó a llorar el / la bebé? **Kwahn**-doh ehm-peh-**soh** ah yoh-**rahr** ehl / lah beh-**beh**?

(X) hours (days, weeks) ago.	(X) horas (días, semanas). (X) **oh**-rahs (**dee**-ahs, seh-**mah**-nahs).
Does he / she bend his / her knees when crying?	¿Dobla las rodillas cuando llora? **Doh**-blah lahs roh-**dee**-yahs **kwahn**-doh **yoh**-rah?
Does the baby cry constantly?	¿Llora el / la bebé constantemente? **Yoh**-rah ehl / lah beh-**beh** kohns-tahn-teh-**mehn**-teh?
Are there periods when the baby stops crying?	¿Hay períodos cuando el / la bebé deja de llorar? **Ah**-ee peh-**ree**-oh-dohs **kwahn**-doh ehl / lah beh-**beh** **deh**-hah deh yoh-**rahr**?
Does he / she cry when he / she urinates (defecates)?	¿Llora cuando orina (obrah / defeca)? **Yoh**-rah **kwahn**-doh oh-**ree**-nah (**oh**-brah / deh-**feh**-kah)?
Is the child constipated?	¿Está estreñido / -a el / la bebé? Ehs-**tah** ehs-treh-**nyee**-doh / -dah ehl / lah beh-**beh**?
Have you noticed blood in his / her stools?	¿Ha notado sangre en sus heces? Ah noh-**tah**-doh **sahn**-greh ehn soos **eh**-sehs?
Does he / she have diarrhea?	¿Tiene diarrea? Tee-**eh**-neh dee-ah-**reh**-ah?
Has he / she been vomiting?	¿Tiene vómito? Tee-**eh**-neh **boh**-mee-toh?
Does he / she have a fever?	¿Tiene fiebre? Tee-**eh**-neh fee-**eh**-breh?

Is he / she pulling his / her ears?	¿Se está tirando o jalando las orejas? Seh ehs-**tah** tee-**rahn**-doh oh hah-**lahn**-doh lahs oh-**reh**-hahs?
Can you console the child?	¿Puede consolar al niño (a la niña)? **Pweh**-deh kohn-soh-**lahr** ahl **nee**-nyoh (ah lah **nee**-nyah)?
Is he / she taking the bottle?	¿Toma la botella? **Toh**-mah lah boh-**teh**-yah?
Have you changed his / her formula?	¿Ha cambiado su fórmula? Ah kahm-bee-**ah**-doh soo **fohr**-moo-lah?
Is he / she teething?	¿Le están saliendo los dientes? Leh ehs-**tahn** sah-lee-**ehn**-doh lohs dee-**ehn**-tehs?

Common Phrases for the Exam for Crying or Colic

Your baby has an ear infection.	Su bebé tiene una infección en el oído. Soo beh-**beh** tee-**eh**-neh oo-nah een-fek-see-**ohn** ehn ehl oh-**ee**-doh.
Your baby has colic.	Su bebé tiene cólico. Soo beh-**beh** tee-**eh**-neh **koh**-lee-koh.
Your baby has a urinary tract infection.	Su bebé tiene una infección de la orina. Soo beh-**beh** tee-**eh**-neh oo-nah een-fek-see-**ohn** deh lah oh-**ree**-nah.

Discharge Instructions for Crying or Colic

Return to the hospital (clinic) if . . .	Regrese al hospital (a la clínica) si... Reh-**greh**-seh ahl ohs-pee-**tahl** (ah lah **klee**-nee-kah) see...
your baby has a fever,	su bebé tiene fiebre, soo beh-**beh** tee-**eh**-neh fee-**eh**-breh,
your baby is vomiting,	su bebé tiene vómito, soo beh-**beh** tee-**eh**-neh **boh**-mee-toh,
there is blood in the baby's stool.	hay sangre en las heces del (de la) bebé. **ah**-ee **sahn**-greh ehn lahs **eh**-sehs dehl (deh lah) beh-**beh**.

Neck Mass

Bola en el Cuello

Boh-lah ehn ehl **kweh**-yoh

How long has there been neck swelling?	¿Cuánto tiempo lleva con la hinchazón en el cuello? **Kwahn**-toh tee-**ehm**-poh yeh-bah kohn lah een-chah-**sohn** ehn ehl **kweh**-yoh?
(X) hours (days, weeks).	(X) horas (días, semanas). (X) **oh**-rahs (**dee**-ahs, seh-**mah**-nahs).
Does he / she have problems swallowing?	¿Tiene problemas al tragar? Tee-**eh**-neh proh-**bleh**-mahs ahl trah-**gahr**?

Does he / she have a fever?	¿Tiene fiebre? Tee-**eh**-neh fee-**eh**-breh?
Does he / she have pain in his / her neck?	¿Tiene dolor en el cuello? Tee-**eh**-neh doh-**lohr** ehn ehl **kweh**-yoh?
Does he / she have pain in his / her ears?	¿Tiene dolor en los oídos? Tee-**eh**-neh doh-**lohr** ehn lohs oh-**ee**-dohs?
Does he / she have pain in his / her teeth?	¿Tiene dolor en los dientes? Tee-**eh**-neh doh-**lohr** ehn lohs dee-**ehn**-tehs?
Does he / she have a sore throat?	¿Tiene dolor de garganta? Tee-**eh**-neh doh-**lohr** deh gahr-**gahn**-tah?
Has he / she had the flu or a cold?	¿Ha tenido gripe o catarro? Ah teh-**nee**-doh gree-peh oh kah-**tah**-roh?
Has he / she lost weight?	¿Ha perdido peso? Ah pehr-**dee**-doh **peh**-soh?
Does he / she have night sweats?	¿Tiene sudores en la noche? Tee-**eh**-neh soo-**doh**-rehs ehn lah **noh**-cheh?
Has he / she been exposed to tuberculosis?	¿Ha sido expuesto / -a a la tuberculosis? Ah **see**-doh eks-**pwehs**-toh / -tah ah lah too-behr-koo-**loh**-sees?
Has he / she taken Tylenol?	¿Ha tomado Tylenol? Ah toh-**mah**-doh **Tay**-leh-nohl?

Common Phrases for the Exam for Neck Mass

I need to take an X ray.	Necesito sacarle una radiografía / unos rayos X. Neh-seh-**see**-toh sah-**kahr**-leh **oo**-nah rah-dee-oh-grah-**fee**-ah / **oo**-nohs **rah**-yohs **eh**-kees.
I need to do a blood test.	Necesito hacerle una prueba de sangre. Neh-seh-**see**-toh ah-**sehr**-leh **oo**-nah **prweh**-bah deh **sahn**-greh.
Your baby has a throat (ear) infection.	Su bebé tiene una infección en la garganta (el oído). Soo beh-**beh** tee-**eh**-neh **oo**-nah een-fek-see-**ohn** ehn lah gahr-**gahn**-tah (ehl oh-**ee**-doh).
Your baby has a tooth abscess.	Su bebé tiene un absceso en el diente. Soo beh-**beh** tee-**eh**-neh oon ab-**seh**-soh ehn ehl dee-**ehn**-teh.

Discharge Instructions for Neck Mass

Give your child his / her medicine (X) times a day.	Dele la medicina a su niño / -a (X) veces al día. **Deh**-leh lah meh-dee-**see**-nah ah soo **nee**-nyoh / -nyah (X) **beh**-sehs ahl **dee**-ah.
Give him / her Tylenol (X) times a day.	Dele Tylenol (X) veces al día. **Deh**-leh **Tay**-leh-nohl (X) **beh**-sehs ahl **dee**-ah.

Return to the hospital (clinic) if . . .	Regrese al hospital (a la clínica) si... Reh-**greh**-seh ahl ohs-pee-**tahl** (ah lah **klee**-nee-kah) see...
your baby has a fever,	su bebé tiene fiebre, soo beh-**beh** tee-**eh**-neh fee-**eh**-breh,
your baby is vomiting,	su bebé tiene vómito, soo beh-**beh** tee-**eh**-neh **boh**-mee-toh,
your baby has difficulty breathing,	su bebé tiene dificultad para respirar, soo beh-**beh** tee-**eh**-neh dee-fee-kool-**tahd pah**-rah rehs-pee-**rahr**,
the neck mass is bigger.	la bola en el cuello crece. lah **boh**-lah ehn ehl **kweh**-yoh **kreh**-seh.

Limp

Cojera

Koh-he-rah

How long has he / she had trouble walking?	¿Cuánto tiempo lleva con dificultad al caminar? **Kwahn**-toh tee-**ehm**-poh **yeh**-bah kohn dee-fee-kool-**tahd** ahl kah-mee-**nahr**?
For (X) hours (days, weeks).	(X) horas (días, semanas). (X) **oh**-rahs (**dee**-ahs, seh-**mah**-nahs).
Did he / she fall?	¿Se cayó? Seh kah-**yoh**?

Did he / she run into something?	¿Se pegó contra algo? Seh peh-**goh kohn**-trah **ahl**-goh?
Does he / she complain of pain in his / her . . .	¿Se queja de dolor en... Seh **keh**-hah deh doh-**lohr** ehn...

	right (left) leg?	la pierna derecha (izquierda)? lah pee-**ehr**-nah deh-**reh**-chah (ees-kee-**ehr**-dah)?
	right (left) knee?	la rodilla derecha (izquierda)? lah roh-**dee**-yah deh-**reh**-chah (ees-kee-**ehr**-dah)?
	right (left) foot?	el pie derecho (izquierdo)? ehl pee-**eh** deh-**reh**-choh (ees-kee-**ehr**-doh)?
	hip?	la cadera? lah kah-**deh**-rah?

Is the area that hurts swollen?	¿Está hinchado donde le duele? Ehs-**tah** een-**chah**-doh **dohn**-deh leh **dweh**-leh?

	Is it red or warm?	¿Está rojo o caliente? Ehs-**tah roh**-hoh oh kah-lee-**ehn**-teh?
	Are other joints swollen?	¿Están hinchadas otras articulaciones? Ehs-**tahn** een-**chah**-dahs **oh**-trahs ahr-tee-koo-lah-see-**oh**-nehs?

Does he / she have bruises?	¿Tiene moretones? Tee-**eh**-neh moh-reh-**toh**-nehs?

Does he / she have a fever?	¿Tiene fiebre? Tee-**eh**-neh fee-**eh**-breh?
Does he / she have a cold?	¿Tiene catarro? Tee-**eh**-neh kah-**tah**-roh?

Common Phrases for the Exam for Limp

I need to take an X ray.	Necesito sacarle una radiografía / unos rayos X. Neh-seh-**see**-toh sah-**kahr**-leh **oo**-nah rah-dee-oh-grah-**fee**-ah / **oo**-nos **rah**-yohs **eh**-kees.
I need to do a blood test.	Necesito hacerle una prueba de sangre. Neh-seh-**see**-toh ah-**sehr**-leh **oo**-nah **prweh**-bah deh **sahn**-greh.
I need to do a bone scan.	Necesito hacerle un escán de los huesos. Neh-seh-**see**-toh ah-**sehr**-leh oon ehs-**kahn** deh lohs **weh**-sohs.
I need to do an ultrasound.	Necesito hacerle un ultrasonido. Neh-seh-**see**-toh ah-**sehr**-leh oon ool-trah-soh-**nee**-doh.
Your baby has an infection in his / her hip (knee).	Su bebé tiene una infección en la cadera (rodilla). Soo beh-**beh** tee-**eh**-neh **oo**-nah een-fek-see-**ohn** ehn lah kah-**deh**-rah (roh-**dee**-yah).
Your baby has a fracture in his / her . . .	Su bebé tiene una fractura en... Soo beh-**beh** tee-**eh**-neh **oo**-nah frak-**too**-rah ehn...

hip.	la cadera. lah kah-**deh**-rah.
right (left) knee.	la rodilla derecha (izquierda). lah roh-**dee**-yah deh-**reh**-chah (ees-kee-**ehr**-dah).
right (left) leg.	la pierna derecha (izquierda). lah pee-**ehr**-nah deh-**reh**-chah (ees-kee-**ehr**-dah).
right (left) ankle.	el tobillo derecho (izquierdo). ehl toh-**bee**-yoh deh-**reh**-choh (ees-kee-**ehr**-doh).

Discharge Instructions for Limp

Give your child his / her medicine (X) times a day.	Dele la medicina a su niño / -a (X) veces al día. **Deh**-leh lah meh-dee-**see**-nah ah soo **nee**-nyoh / -nyah (X) **beh**-sehs ahl **dee**-ah.
Give him / her Tylenol (X) times a day.	Dele Tylenol (X) veces al día. **Deh**-leh **Tay**-leh-nohl (X) **beh**-sehs ahl **dee**-ah.
Return to the hospital (clinic) if . . .	Regrese al hospital (a la clínica) si... Reh-**greh**-seh ahl ohs-pee-**tahl** (ah lah **klee**-nee-kah) see...
your baby (still) has a fever,	su bebé (todavía) tiene fiebre, soo beh-**beh** (toh-dah-**bee**-ah) tee-**eh**-neh fee-**eh**-breh,

your baby still has
difficulty walking
(moving),

su bebé todavía tiene
dificultad para caminar
(moverse),
soo beh-**beh** toh-dah-**bee**-
ah tee-**eh**-neh dee-fee-
kool-**tahd pah**-rah kah-
mee-**nahr** (moh-**behr**-seh),

the swelling is worse.

la hinchazón está peor.
lah een-chah-**sohn** ehs-**tah**
peh-**ohr**.

Appendix: Pronunciation

In Spanish, the letters are pronounced similar to those in English, with the exception of the letters listed below.

a   sounds like a clipped "ah," as in *father.*
     aborto (*abortion*) = ah-**bohr**-toh
     cama (*bed*) = **kah**-mah

b   sounds like "b" in book.
     brazo (*arm*) = **brah**-soh
     boca (*mouth*) = **boh**-kah

c   before **a**, **o**, **u**, or a consonant has a hard "k" sound.
     calambre (*cramp*) = kah-**lahm**-breh, **cuello** (*neck*) =
     kweh-yoh, **clínica** (*clinic*) = **klee**-nee-kah
     before **e** or **i** has a soft *s* sound.
     medicina (*medicine*) = meh-dee-**see**-nah
     cerebro (*brain*) = seh-**reh**-broh

e   sounds like "eh" as in *bed.*
     pecho (*chest*) = **peh**-choh
     estómago (*stomach*) = ehs-**toh**-mah-goh

g   before **a**, **o**, **u**, or a consonant has a hard sound (as in *get*).
     garganta (*throat*) = gahr-**gahn**-tah
     goteo (*drip*) = goh-**teh**-oh
     before **e** or *i* has a soft *h* sound.
     vagina (*vagina*) = vah-**hee**-nah
     alergia (*allergy*) = ah-**lehr**-hee-ah

h   is always silent.
     hospital (*hospital*) = ohs-pee-**tahl**
     inhalar (*to inhale*) = een-ah-**lahr**

i   sounds like the "ee" in *meet.*
     infarto (*infarct*) = een-**fahr**-toh
     infección (*infection*) = een-fek-see-**ohn**

j	sounds like the English "h."

ojo (*eye*) = **oh**-hoh
mejilla (*cheek*) = meh-**hee**-yah

ll	sounds like the "y" in *yes* or *you*.

tobillo (*ankle*) = toh-**bee**-yoh
llaga (*sore*) = **yah**-gah

ñ	sounds like the English "ny" in *canyon* or the "ni" in *onion*.

riñón (*kidney*) = ree-**nyohn**
estreñimiento (*constipation*) = ehs-treh-nyee-mee-**ehn**-toh

o	sounds like "oh," as in *low*.

operación (*operation*) = oh-pee-rah-see-**ohn**
orina (*urine*) = oh-**ree**-nah

qu	has a "k" sound (the **u** is silent).

quijada (*jaw*) = kee-**hah**-dah
bronquitis (*bronchitis*) = brohn-**kee**-tees

rr	pronounce it with a hard roll like the commercial "Ruffles have ridges."

gonorrea (*gonorrhea*) = goh-noh-**rheh**-ah
catarro (*cold*) = kah-**tah**-rhoh

u	sounds like "ooh," as in *do*.

úvula (*uvula*) = **oo**-boo-lah
usted (*you*) = oos-**tehd**
before a vowel, it usually sounds like the English "w," as in *twang*.
duerme (*sleep*) = **dwehr**-meh
fue (*was*) = fweh

v	sounds like the English "b."

vesícula (*gallbladder*) = beh-**see**-koo-lah
vena (*vein*) = **beh**-nah

y   sounds like the English "y" in yes.
    yeso (*cast*) = yeh-**soh**
    sounds like "j" in judge if the "y" follows "n."
    inyección (*injection*) = een-**jeg**-see-ohn

z   sounds like the English "s."
    corazón (*heart*) = koh-rah-**sohn**
    embarazada (*pregnant*) = ehm-bah-rah-**sah**-dah

Index